IT'S PARKINSON'S...

A DAUGHTER'S JOURNEY THROUGH PARKINSON'S WITH HER MOTHER

CARYN MEARS

outskirts press

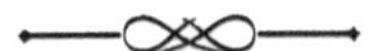

Dedicated to my mother,
who allowed me to join her on her journey through Parkinson's;
and to my sisters, Cathy and Lann, and my step-brother, Bruce,
who supported me as we muddled through
these unnavigated waters together.
There were times when our canoe felt like it was upside down;
but we managed to bring it upright and stay the course.
Thank you for being there with me.

TABLE OF CONTENTS

CHAPTER 1

THE DOCTOR'S VISIT

"IT'S PARKINSONS," SAID the doctor, his gentle hand holding my mother's tiny wrinkled hand cupped in his. Mom and I sat rigidly perched on our chairs, like two old crows sitting frozen on a high wire in the middle of winter. It was as if we were suspended in time, not knowing what to say, or how to react. Mom's eyes seemed to glaze over, as if she was staring into the unknown, and instinctively, I could tell without her saying a word, that her mind was somewhere else.

"You have Akinetic Rigid Parkinson's, which means your body wants to freeze," the doctor was saying. His voice again was kind and soft, filled with compassion as he went on, "I'm afraid there is no medication that can help you with this kind of Parkinson's." He stopped and then added, "Do you have any questions?"

"Questions?" Mom asked, still stunned with this new information. The silence swarming around us was deafening. Mom cleared her throat. In her weak voice she whispered, "What kind of Parkinson's did you say I have?" Her voice, feeble with age, giving away her eighty-four years. Mom wanted to know exactly what she was dealing with so she could do research on this new disease.

"Akinetic Rigid Parkinson's," the doctor repeated slowly. "Akinetic means you will have moments where your body won't move, and of course, rigid means your body will freeze. It's as if your brain forgets to tell your body what to do, and your muscles stop working."

"You could tell that just by watching me walk across the room?" Mom asked, motioning her hand across the room where she had just walked. Connie was a petite woman with meticulously quaffed white hair. She barely weighed ninety pounds and stood at just four feet ten inches tall, having shrunk significantly from her once five foot, two frame. She'd been a dancer, and as she shuffled across the exam room for Dr. German, there was no evidence of her once graceful ballroom moves. No tango steps entered her shuffle as Dr. German and his nurse watched her muddle her way along the side of the exam table crossing the five foot expanse of the tiny exam room. With her cane by her side, she strategically turned and managed her way back to her chair where she collapsed. In that small feat, Dr. German, the most sought after neurologist in Las Vegas, diagnosed her with her worst fear.

"Yes, I could tell from your walk," he nodded, adding, "it's Parkinson's, but I'd like you to come in for more testing next week."

"Will I be able to use my walker?" Mom asked, looking up at the doctor. The sparkle had faded from her usual laughing eyes as she reached for her walker, the one piece of medical equipment she relied on the most.

"Yes, you can still use your walker, but you'll need to put some tennis balls on the back of this one," he said. "Having tennis balls on the back will help keep you from falling backwards," he told her. "That's a serious problem for people with Parkinson's," he went on. "We don't want you to fall backwards." Mom seemed to soak that information in as her gaze went towards the window.

I wondered, "What was she thinking?"

"I'll let you sit here for a moment," said the doctor, "and when you're ready, you can go out to the front desk and make another appointment for further testing." He stood up, followed by his nurse, who had been sitting next to him in the small exam room. They both stepped sideways to maneuver around Mom's walker, inching their way to the door. They appeared eager to make their exit, having just delivered disastrous news to yet another patient. Looking back over her shoulder, the nurse's eyes were filled with compassion for the fragile women left sitting with her daughter in the exam room. Delivering this diagnosis was never easy.

Mom sighed. Reaching for her walker, she struggled to place her purse into the pocket of the walker. A red cardinal applique had been glued onto the pocket of the walker. My youngest sister had gotten Mom the red walker for Christmas, and my other sister had added the cardinal as a loving touch. It helped distinguish Mom's walker from the myriad of others in the dining hall at her retirement facility. With great effort, Mom pressed her hands against the walker and raised her body out of the chair. Her arms were still strong, and they strained as she lifted her body with amazing determination. I moved over to the door, opening it wide. Once standing erect, Mom started her shuffle out of the exam room and down the long corridor to the appointment desk. With her eyes staring straight ahead, she refused to let the tears fall. She was a strong stoic woman and had faced many trials and tribulations in her life. She would bear this one, too, whatever it was going to bring her way.

Quickly getting in front of Mom, I said, "This way," motioning her towards a different hallway from the one we had entered.

"But didn't we come in this way?" she asked, looking confused.

"You're right." I said. "We came in down that hall, but this is the way they want us to leave. We have to go make another appointment. I guess it's like Chaparral Pet Clinic," I told her. "They have one way in and another way out," I explained. She and my step-father, a veterinarian, had built their own clinic in Las Vegas many years earlier, and I hoped the analogy would help her understand the going into and going out of the neurologists clinic. The look of confusion on her face as she pursed her lips told me she truly wasn't understanding, but she was complying to my wishes.

Once we reached the appointment desk, the lady behind the counter looked at me and said, "We can get you in next week at the same time, will that be okay?"

"That will be fine," I said, as I reached across the counter to take the reminder card.

As we shuffled slowly around the corner, Mom discovered we were back at the main lobby where we had entered the clinic. "Now this is where we came in," she said, with a slight smile starting to spread across her face as a sense of familiarity eased her mind.

"You're right," I said, "and now we just have to get to the car!" I led Mom through the large doors of the building. Her slow shuffle seemed to take longer than when we first transitioned into the building. Mom needed help getting the walker over the threshold of the door and even the cracks in the sidewalk appeared to be challenges. Stepping down the curb presented a new obstacle as we approached the car. I took Mom's arm and guided her closer to the car. I lifted her walker down the curb. Mom followed. First one foot and then the other. Opening the passenger door, I eased Mom around the open door and helped her, backside first, into the passenger seat. "I wonder if anyone has invented a swivel seat," I said to myself. Lifting her legs up over the threshold of the car door, I swung them around to the front of the passenger seat. Leaning over Mom, I buckled her seatbelt. Grabbing the large walker, I took it to the back of the car, where I opened the rear door of her Rav 4, folded the walker, and laid it inside. As I walked around to the driver's door and slid behind the steering wheel, I was exhausted. Letting out a huge sigh, I thought to myself, "It's almost like having a toddler again."

I turned the key in the ignition, and it felt odd driving Mom's car. She had always been the one to drive me around when I visited Las Vegas. She knew all of the shortcuts, but now our roles were reversed.

"I'm going to take the freeway home," I told her, adding, "It's faster for me, avoiding all the stop lights on Eastern." Mom was too exhausted to argue. She had gotten up at her usual 4:30 in the morning to have a cup of coffee; and watch the sunrise over the mountains. She had done her morning crossword puzzle; and had gotten ready for her doctor's appointment. These days, just getting dressed was an effort. She had lived alone for twenty-five years since my step-father had passed away. She had been a very independent woman until I insisted she get someone to help her with mowing the lawn and cleaning the pool. She had done it all: the mowing, the roses, and the cleaning of the swimming pool, but now I had to physically help her into her own car as if she were a toddler. I knew she was exhausted, and all she had done was visit the doctor.

Turning on the air conditioner to combat the Las Vegas heat, I could tell Mom was deep in thought, but all of a sudden she interrupted my thoughts. "Miss Independent is gonna' need some help!" she said. "What am I going to do if I can't drive? Who will get my groceries?" The worry in her voice was evident.

"We'll all help you," I said, "but maybe it's time we get you some extra help." I stopped and looked at her, and then turned back keeping my eyes on the road.

"I've already experienced the freezing the doctor was talking about," she said quietly.

"You have?" I gasped. "What happened?"

"One night I was walking to dinner, going across the large courtyard on my way to the dining hall, and my legs just stopped working," she explained. "I couldn't go forward or backwards. I was frozen."

"What did you do?" My voice rose to a higher pitch, alarmed as I asked her this question. I was picturing my eighty-four year old mother frozen like a statue in the middle of all the buildings surrounding the courtyard.

"I just stood there." she said. "Right in the middle of the courtyard. I kept telling my legs to walk, but they wouldn't move."

"That must have been scary," I said, as I signaled to turn right onto Eastern Blvd. "What did you do next?" I asked.

"What could I do?" she said. "I waited a minute or two, but it seemed like an eternity. I had no idea how long it would take to get my feet to work again," she said, her voice almost a whisper.

"Wow, you couldn't even yell out for help," I said. "Your voice isn't very loud anymore."

"I don't know how long I stood there, but all of a sudden one foot stepped forward and I was walking again. It was the strangest thing, " she said, staring out the window, thinking about her endeavor.

Putting two and two together, I realized Akinetic Rigid Parkinson's had presented itself. "I think we need to get someone to help you get to dinner," I said. "You have the longest walk to the dining room of anyone who lives in your apartment building."

"Yes," said Mom, "my body just didn't want to cooperate anymore. I kept telling myself just one step forward, but nothing would move, and then all of a sudden, as if by some miraculous intervention, my foot stepped forward."

"That must have been so scary," I said again, looking over at her.

"It sure was!" said Mom. "Now, when I'm walking, I constantly say to myself 'left, right, left, right'. I really have to concentrate. I don't want to freeze again! It was very scary."

"Not to mention, frustrating," I said, as we drove on in silence, both of us lost in our own thoughts.

Mom sighed, "Eighty-four years old!" she said quietly, exasperated from the morning's ordeal. "Why would I get this Parkinson's at eighty-four years old? I've lived my whole life. Why would I get it now?" she asked as she plunked her hands in her lap in total frustration.

"Well, it's a lot better than getting it at sixty-four!" I joked, trying to lighten the mood, but Mom didn't think I was funny.

"Where is Bill when I need him the most?" she said mournfully, thinking of her husband who had passed away twenty five years earlier. "He was supposed to be the one to take care of me!" she said feeling sorry for herself.

"I know," I said with as much empathy as I could muster. "It doesn't seem fair. I wish he were here, too. It would have been nice if he could have outlived you, instead of the other way around."

Lost in our own thoughts, Mom thinking about her future and missing her late husband, and me wondering who I could call for elder care. We had been introduced to Parkinson's, and it wasn't going to affect just one of us. It was going to affect the entire family.

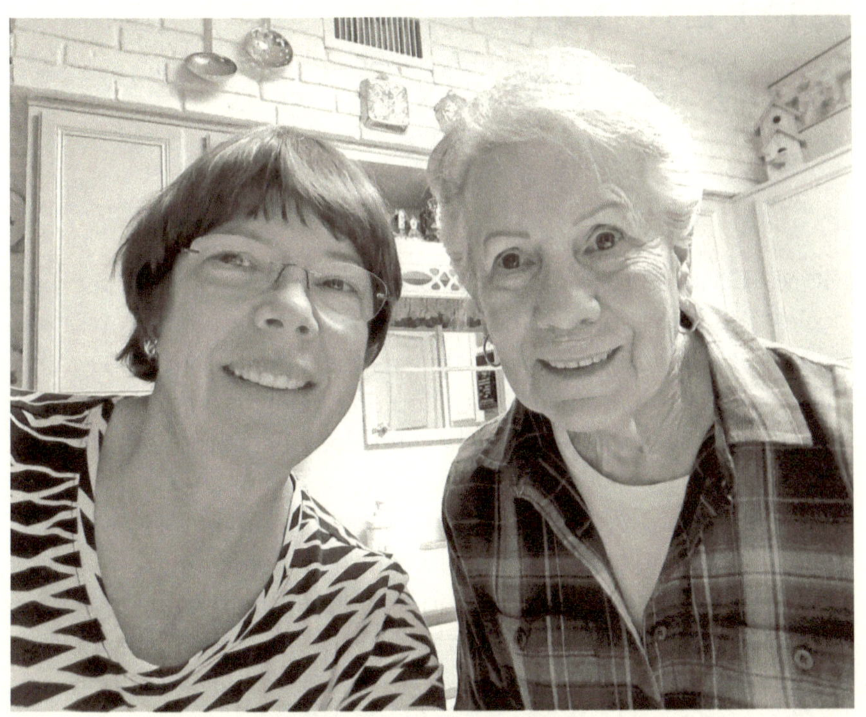

Author Caryn Mears showing her mother,
Connie Mears, about selfies, 2018.

CHAPTER 2

AFTER THE APPOINTMENT

MOM ADMITTED THAT she had been afraid this would be her diagnosis. "I've been doing some research based on my symptoms," she said, "but when I heard the doctor say the actual word, Parkinson's, I felt like I was in a dream. I just couldn't believe it. I had prayed so hard not to hear that word," she said, looking at me with her sad brown eyes.

I nodded my head. "It was still a shock, when that was what you were anticipating, wasn't it?" I said, affirming her feelings.

She nodded, no longer able to talk about her ordeal. My petite, white haired mother was an incredibly strong individual, and although she had presented a strong demeanor in the exam room, she had been crushed by that one single word; Parkinson's.

As a walking medical encyclopedia, Mom had always been able to provide us with answers or guidance for any of our medical questions. Whenever my sister, Cathy, needed medical advice, Mom was the person she would call for a quick answer. If Mom didn't know the answer, she knew exactly where to find it in her plethora of medical books. Mom was giving medical advice long before the internet was even a thing, so days before her appointment with Dr, German, the neurologist, she looked up her symptoms and basically diagnosed herself.

"Parkinson's," she said. "My research said I had Parkinson's, but when I heard the doctor say it outloud, it felt like a death sentence," she said. "I had been mentally preparing for the diagnosis, but it still knocked me for a loop."

"It seems like Parkinson's is becoming more common. Isn't that the disease where old people shake?" I asked.

"But I'm not shaking," Mom said, "which makes it very perplexing, and I don't ever want to be one of those people whose head wobbles to and fro." She had seen others with hands quivering, or limbs uncontrollably shaking, and she did not want her body doing that. She was a person who was always in control, and she definitely wanted to be in control of her own body. "I'm not going to let this disease control me," she said, trying to be emphatic by again putting her hands in her lap, but her voice was becoming almost a whisper.

Living in Las Vegas since 1972, Mom loved the desert. Unfortunately, I was living in Washington state, a sixteen hour drive away, or a two hour flight on Allegiant Airlines. Both of us were deep in thought trying to imagine our futures as we entered the parking lot of The Echelon, the senior living residence Mom had chosen when she needed to sell her house. She had only been living at the Echelon for just a few months when we were finally able to get her a doctor's appointment.

As I pulled the car into the parking stall, I turned off the engine and opened my door. "We're home," I announced and headed to the back of the car where I retrieved the walker and brought it around to Mom's side of the car. Opening the passenger door, I reached in and unbuckled Mom's seatbelt. Our faces were so close I could have kissed her. I should have hugged her. I kick myself now for not taking that opportunity. God knows she could have used a hug, but instead I proceeded to put the seatbelt back, reach down and grab her legs, swinging her feet around to her side so her legs were dangling out of the car. I was all business as I struggled to help lift her to a standing position. Reaching around, I grabbed the walker and rolled it in front of Mom. "There, we go," I said as we shuffled over to the sidewalk. Mom could handle the short walk to her apartment as I quickly went back to close the car door and lock it. Following her down the sidewalk, I secretly video-taped her slow shuffle. Then I quickly raced around her snail-paced speed, and got in front of her to unlock her apartment door.

"The sun is shining and it's so beautiful here," I thought as I put the key into the lock and opened the door. "It's another day in paradise," I said, mimicking what my step father used to say as I swung the door open, and helped Mom across the threshold with her walker. She set her purse on the credenza by the door, and made her way a few more steps to her recliner. She literally collapsed into her recliner before she was even lined up to sit down properly.

I had purchased the recliner as a present for her, telling her it was purchased by my son. It was the kind of chair that raises you up to a standing position, and Mom was enamored with the coziness it offered. She let out a sigh, "Oh, it's good to be home, but I'm so hungry!" she said.

"Exhausted and starving," I said as I put together her standard lunch, a small bowl of peaches with a spoon, and a rice cracker with a jar of peanut butter, and a knife. Putting everything on a tray, I took it to her while she sat in her chair, not wanting her to get up. I knew she was exhausted.

"This is service," she said, and smiled. We began chatting about our morning expedition.

"I know you're tired," I said, "but just look at how far you've come over the past twenty five years. You can be so proud of yourself: living alone, selling your house, and moving into this place."

"We bought that house in 1977," Mom said, "and now it is 2018. I lived there for over forty years."

"I remember," I told her. "You hosted our wedding reception at your new house on Seneca Drive in 1977. We were so lucky to have that beautiful pool and the atrium as a backdrop for the reception. You were quite the little Energizer Bunny in those days: cleaning the pool, taking care of the yard, and working at the clinic!" I told her, remembering those long ago days.

"Yes, and I did that for almost the entire time I lived there, until you forced me to get a gardener and a poolman!" she said.

As an elderly woman, Mom ran out of money, and had to sell her house in order to have money to live on. Her estate sale had been a farce, getting only pennies for what she had paid thousands of dollars for during her lifetime, but she knew it was something she had to do. It was difficult for her to part with her magnificent furniture, grand piano and artwork, but in the long run, it was worth it. Fortunately, she was allowed to bring many of her prized possessions with her to The Echelon, including her violin which she had played in Wayne Newton's orchestra.

"Now, everything is done for you. You have someone to cook your meals, vacuum, and dust. They'll even change your sheets if you ask them," I said. "I wish I could live here with you!" I joked, which finally brought a smirk to her face.

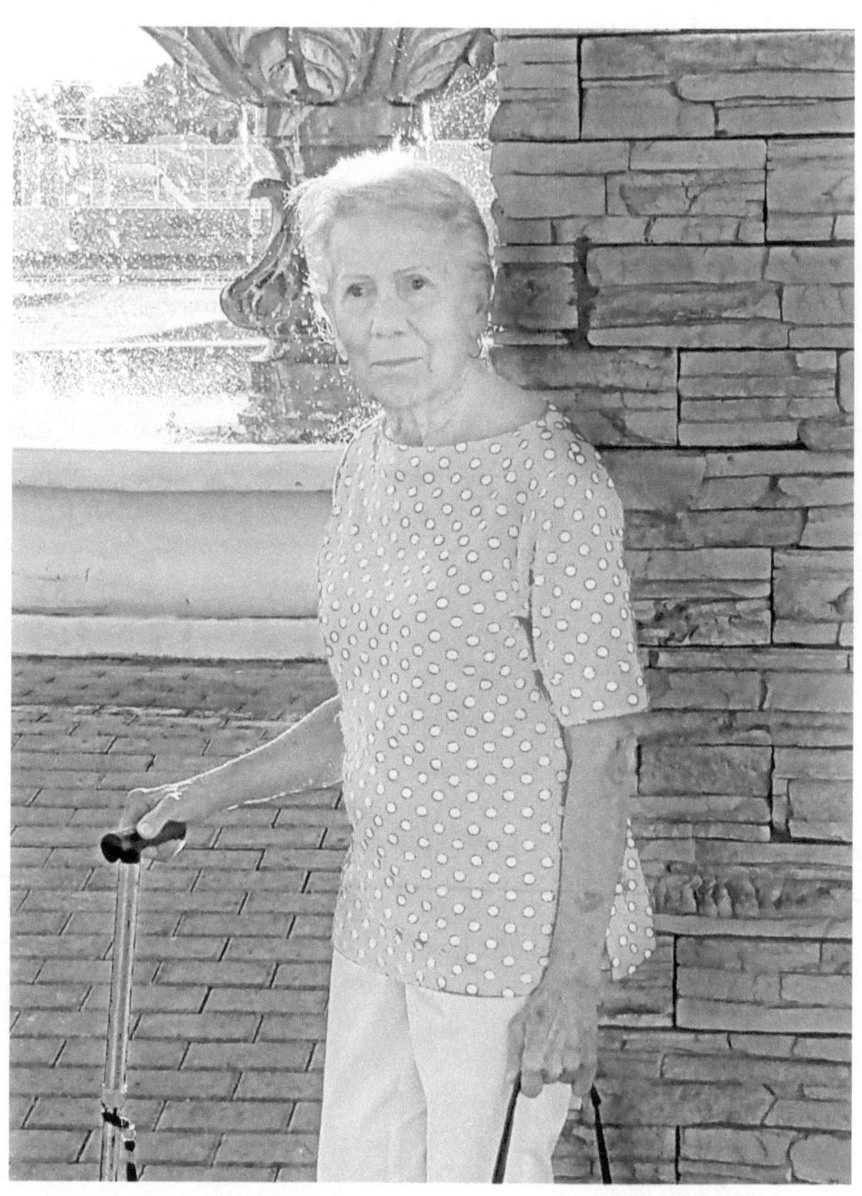

Mom at The Echelon Senior Living Community

CHAPTER 3

CALLING HER CHILDREN

WALKING OVER TO Mom's computer, I pulled out the chair and turned on her antiquated machine. It was positioned on a desk allowing the user to look directly out through the large bay window onto the courtyard. I had a panoramic view of the courtyard where Mom had faced her Akinetic Rigid Parkinson's freezing episode. I shook my head, as if clearing the cobwebs from my brain, imagining how frightened she must have been standing in the middle of that large area with no one around to help her.

When the computer finally lit up, I googled 'Akinetic Rigid Parkinson's,' but I soon discovered there was a limited amount of information about Mom's specific type of Parkinson's available online. I did, however, learn about Parkinson's in general. According to the American Parkinson's Disease Association, "Parkinson's is a type of movement disorder that can affect the ability to perform common, daily activities." I went on to read that "Parkinson's is a chronic and progressive disease where symptoms become worse over time. It is characterized by its most common motor symptoms, tremors, a form of rhythmic shaking, stiffness or rigidity of muscles, and slowness of movement, but it also manifests in non-motor symptoms including sleep problems, constipation, anxiety, depression and fatigue."

"What did you find out?" asked Mom, looking up from the book she was reading.

"Well, there isn't much on the internet about your specific kind of Parkinson's." I said. What I didn't tell my mother was that her journey wasn't going to be easy by any means. Just as Mom's gait was beginning to freeze, I learned that her non-motor functions would also begin to freeze. Her swallowing reflexes would cease, or her lungs would freeze, or even her heart would forget to keep beating. Choking and pneumonia were listed as the main causes of death, and none of the other outcomes proved to be pleasant possibilities.

As I shut down the computer and walked back to the sofa to sit closer to Mom's recliner, I noticed her lunch tray was finished and I picked it up and took it back to the kitchen. "I think we should call Lann and Cathy," I told Mom, walking back to sit on the sofa. Getting my cell phone out of my pocket, I said, "They're probably waiting to find out the results of your doctor's visit this morning."

Together, Mom and I explained to my sisters, Cathy in Minnesota, and Lann in San Francisco, what had transpired in Dr. German's office. As we expected, they had both been waiting to hear what the doctor had to say.

I explained to each one individually as I held the phone out for Mom and I to both be able to speak. "The doctor had Mom walk across the exam room with her cane, and when she sat down, he very politely took her hand and said, 'It's Parkinson's.'"

"He said that it's the kind of Parkinson's that doesn't have any medication that will help," Mom added.

"Yes," I said. "Her kind of Parkinson's is called 'Akinetic Rigid Parkinsons', and it is a type of Parkinson's where your body freezes. That's why we haven't seen her shake much," I explained that it's mostly about the freezing.

"What are they going to do for you?" asked Cathy.

"They want to do more tests, so we have another appointment next week." I said, "However, I'm not sure why. They already gave us a diagnosis."

"Growing old isn't for sissies!" Mom interjected, trying to throw some lightheartedness into the scene. "Parkinson's," she sighed, "who would have thought this would be my demise?"

"Well, at least you still have your sense of humor!" said Cathy, and the three women laughed together.

"That's for sure." said Mom. "You need to have a sense of humor to survive this life." Mom sighed and ran her finger across her neck, signaling to me she was done talking on the phone.

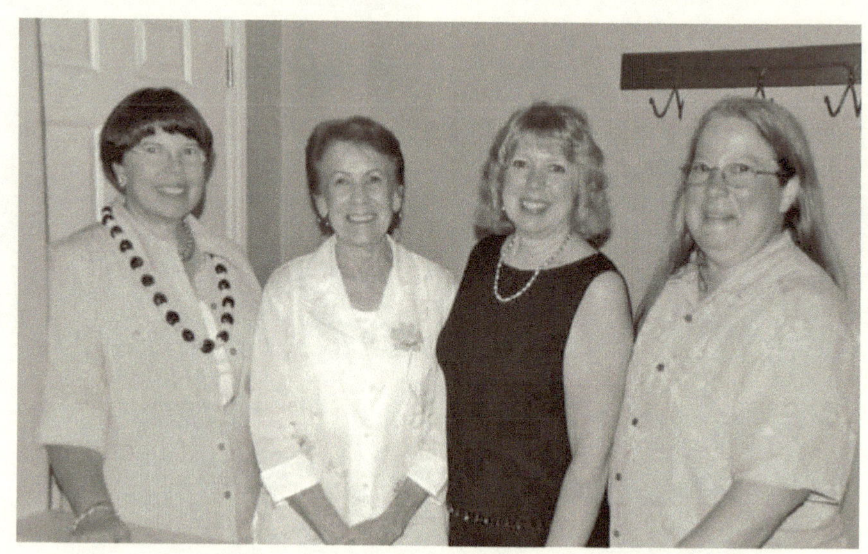

Mom, in white, with author Caryn Mears, and her sisters, Cathy Peterson and Lann Wilder.

CHAPTER **4**

WHAT IS PARKINSON'S?

ONCE WE FINISHED our conversation with Cathy, we called Lann, and then Mom began to doze. I shifted my position on the couch, reaching for the small plastic sack of goodies we had received from the doctor's office. I took out a small booklet called, <u>A Parkinson's Disease Handbook, A Guide for Patients and Their Families'</u> by Lawrence I Gotbe, Margery H. Mark and Jacob I. Sage. "I might as well get comfortable," I thought, as I kicked my shoes off and stretched my legs up onto the large oak coffee table in front of the sofa. There, nestled against the pillow, with my feet comfortably propped on the coffee table, I began to learn about this new disease.

"Parkinson's is a progressive disease of the brain," I read.

"Well, this isn't new to me," I thought, having just read the same information during my Google search, but for some reason it hit me smack dab in the face. Mom has a disease that is affecting her brain. She'd always been an avid reader with a phenomenal vocabulary; quick with accounting; and physically very active. In her younger days she had played softball, run hurdles in track, and was the Iowa State Women's Freestyle Archery Champion, not to mention, she played piano, violin and organ. I couldn't imagine Mom slowing down. She still loved doing her crossword puzzles and walking every day.

"In healthy brains, cells called neurons make a chemical called dopamine, and that chemical coordinates the body's movements."

I read straight out of the booklet, "People who are diagnosed with Parkinson's have too little dopamine in their brains, and their neurons begin to die."

"That's what's happening to Mom." I thought. "Her brain is dying, and the lack of dopamine is slowing her movements." I looked over at my mother. Her head was slumped, her chin nearly touching her chest. She was peacefully sleeping in her recliner, totally unaware of what was happening inside her body. "Low dopamine levels cause tremors, slow movement and problems with balance," said the booklet.

"So this is what happens when the dopamine levels drop," I thought to myself, "and it's exactly what's happening to Mom right now!" It was as if the article had been written specifically for her.

The "eighty-year old shuffle" Mom displayed as she walked across the doctor's office was something she couldn't control. It was Parkinson's, and the lack of dopamine forced her into this festinating gait, meaning she was taking small, rapid steps in a forward motion while trying to keep her body upright. That's what the doctor had seen. All this time I thought her shuffling was a sign of aging, but when I watched others around her who were even older, I didn't notice them shuffling. Now, reading about Parkinson's and the lack of dopamine, I realized, Mom's balance and gait were caused by a lack of dopamine in her brain.

"That's it!" I said to myself. "Mom just needs more dopamine. I found the answer to her problem." However, then I remembered Dr. German specifically explaining there were no medical treatments for Mom's type of Parkinson's. That's when I read, "Medical treatments can only manage the symptoms. There is no cure."

As Mom stirred, trying to shift positions in her recliner, I read about the early symptoms of the disease. Some people have gastrointestinal difficulties, like constipation, because the intestines have difficulty moving food through the system. Mom had mentioned that she had been constipated a little more than usual. In her sixties, I remember her making a beeline to the bathroom in the morning, but now she often said, "I had to work it out with a pencil," while her bowel movement made an appearance.

Next I read, "Some people lose their sense of smell." Mom hadn't mentioned losing her sense of smell, but living alone for so long, none of us knew what she was truly experiencing unless she mentioned it.

The booklet stated, "Parkinson patients may have sleep disorders such as insomnia, restless leg syndrome, or excessive daytime sleepiness." Again, living so far away, I had no idea whether Mom had experienced these symptoms, although I do know one of her doctor's had prescribed a glass of wine at night to help her get to sleep.

A few years earlier, Cathy and I had noticed Mom's handwriting becoming extremely small. If only we had known that this micrographia was a symptom of Parkinson's. Her handwriting had always consisted of large swirling strokes, but as I watched her sign the paperwork for the sale of her house, I noticed how difficult it was for her to make her writing legible. It was at this same time that Cathy noticed Mom was struggling to keep her checkbook and household expenses in order. Little did we know these were also beginning symptoms of Parkinson's.

We had also noticed a small tremor in Mom's pointer finger, but she dismissed it as a sign of aging. "It's hell to grow old!" she had said. Living so far away and seeing her only once or twice a year, we dismissed her ailments as a part of the aging process. After all, Mom was our medical aficionado! She knew everything medical. She couldn't have anything wrong with her!

Through those few years when Mom was growing old, we discovered she was experiencing several slips, trips and falls. I had chastised her one afternoon when she told me about her fall from the ladder.

"What were you doing up on a ladder?" I asked.

"I was just doing a little touch up painting along the patio gutters," she had explained. "I'm only going up one step," she said, trying to assuage my fears.

"I don't want you going up even one step," I sternly admonished her. "Eighty year old ladies shouldn't be on ladders." I could tell Mom was smiling on the other end of the phone.

Another day Mom called to inform me she had tripped on the cord to the blinds in the den. "I was just adjusting the window blinds, and when I walked away, I caught my foot on the cord," she said. "I have a huge bruise on my arm and my leg," she added. Another phone call resulted in her catching her leg on the dining room table, falling and creating yet more bruises.

"You're a walking catastrophe," I said, "but at least you're moving."

"I have to keep moving," she said, "the alternative isn't that great!"

Her next fall proved to be more serious than we realized and she wasn't even moving around. Mom had been in the midst of selling her house, and she was going to be showing it to a prospective buyer the next day. While on the phone with me, she described her latest fall.

"I don't know what happened," she said, "I had to get up in the middle of the night to pee. It was the strangest thing because I never have to do that."

"Well, you're lucky," I said. "Sometimes I have to get up twice a night," I joked.

"This was different. I don't know what happened. I was sitting on the toilet peeing and peeing. It was like I couldn't turn the faucet off. It just wouldn't stop, and all of a sudden I woke up on the floor in a pool of blood. I think I fell asleep on the toilet and then hit my head on the floor when I fell."

"Oh my gosh!" I gasped, "Did you go to the emergency room? You need to get checked out!" I said, wondering what I could do from Washington state.

"It's okay," she explained. "I went into the emergency room, and they x-rayed my head. They were concerned about a concussion, and I ended up having one," she said, "and several stitches." She was very matter of fact as she described this traumatic experience!

"What time did this happen?" I asked.

"It was about 3:00 in the morning, but I had to get everything cleaned up so I could show the house later that afternoon. It looked like there had been a murder in the bathroom," she explained, "so I had to get a bunch of towels and clean up the blood.

"You waited until three in the afternoon to go to the emergency room?" I asked.

"Well, I had to show the house first," Mom explained.

"Oh my gosh! You could have called the real estate agent and told them to come earlier or later. You could have even canceled," I told her. Mom remained cool, calm and collected. She had taken care of everything herself. She was in control.

Now, I was looking back at that incident, and wondering if Mom had actually had a stroke. The emergency room hadn't checked for a stroke. Instead they completed x-rays to check for a concussion which they discovered, or maybe they discovered she had a stroke and didn't tell her. Her slips, trips, and falls were indicative of Parkinson's. We had missed all of the other signs because we didn't know we were looking for Parkinson's. In hindsight, the timing of this fall seemed to indicate Parkinson's was alive and well in Mom's body. Unfortunately, I was totally unaware of this silent disease creeping into Mom's life like a prowler, robbing her of her abilities to maneuver through life. .

Turning the page in the booklet, I read "The Five Stages of Parkinson's." The first stage described one-sided motor symptoms, such as a tremor in one hand or stiffness in one leg, and then I remembered Mom's pointer finger trembling. We had missed that symptom. During the first stage, some people have changes in their posture or facial expressions, but there is very little impact on mobility. We had definitely missed that first stage due to living so far away.

"In Stage 2, motor symptoms are affected on both sides of the body, and daily tasks, such as getting dressed, may take longer." Mom had mentioned that getting dressed was taking her much longer, but we again addressed that slowness as part of her injuries or the aging process.

"Problems with speech and posture may also appear at this stage," the booklet said. I remembered Mom's slurred speech. We had attributed it to her new dental problems, but we had actually missed another symptom. It dawned on me that Mom had passed through stage one and stage two without us even noticing.

"In Stage 3 balance is affected, and daily tasks are more difficult," I read, and I wondered if this was the stage Mom was in now, but then I read about the next stage. "In Stage 4 symptoms are so bad that a person will need help with daily tasks such as brushing their teeth, fixing meals, et. They may not be able to live alone."

"Bingo!" I said out loud, causing Mom to stir, and then I thought to myself. "This is probably the stage Mom is at right now." Although Mom had been able to get up on her own in the morning, get her morning paper at the front door, make her own breakfast and lunch, and get back and forth to the bathroom on her own, she was struggling to get to the dining hall for her evening meals. It was literally a quarter of a mile long walk over to the dining hall. That's when it dawned on me, we not only missed Stages 1 and 2, but we'd also missed Stage 3, and we were now dealing with Stages 4-5.

"In stage 4, falling is a major risk and getting in and out of bed is difficult. A Parkinson's patient may need a wheelchair in Stage 5." That's when I understood, Mom was going to need lots of help.

Along with very slight tremors, rigid freezing, and her impaired balance, Mom was dealing with other symptoms. She was experiencing slowness in her walking, and showing the typical Parkinson's gait. Bradykinesia is a slowness of movement as well as the complete loss of movement, or freezing. She wasn't swinging her arms when she walked, but I thought it was because she was using a cane. She was also showing signs of decreased facial muscles and decreased blinking. Her vision was becoming a problem as she struggled with her daily crossword puzzle, let alone reading her own chicken scratching. Mom was already experiencing slurred speech, but hadn't realized it, and her voice had softened to the point where she was almost whispering. Her posture was stooped as she shuffled along with her walker.

Now it was my job to help Mom adapt to the shock of her diagnosis, and help her deal with the grief that accompanies this disabling disease called Parkinson's.

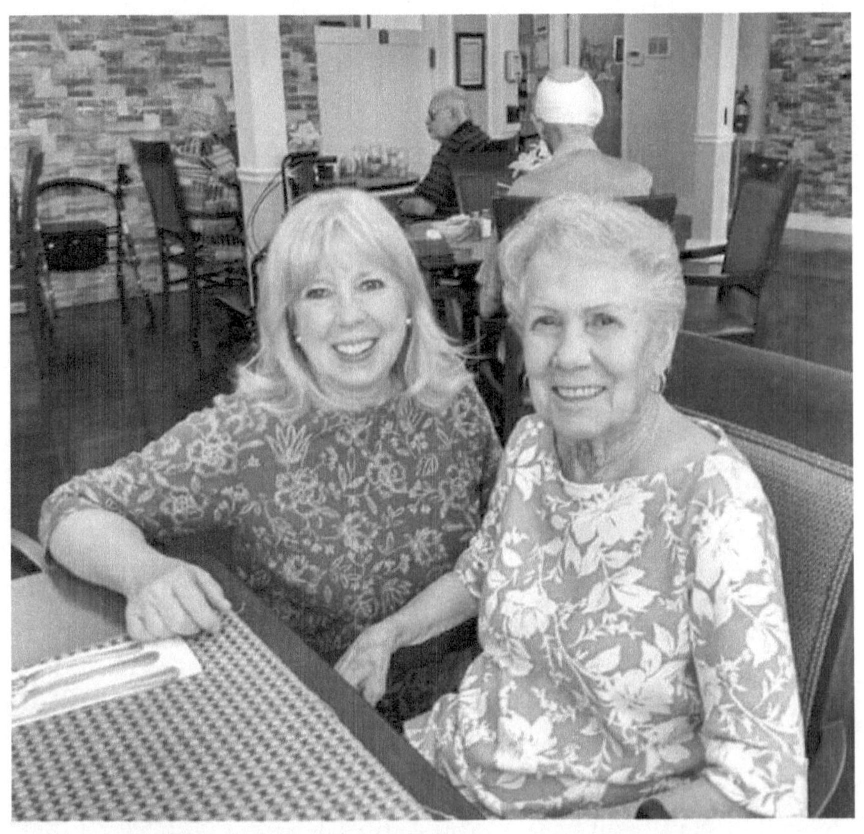

Mom enjoying the dining room at The Echelon Senior Living Community with daughter, Cathy Peterson.

CHAPTER 5

LIFE BEFORE PARKINSON'S

IT WAS MARCH,1977, when Mom and Bill Mears purchased their thirty-two hundred square foot house located at 3398 Seneca Drive. Their lovely home, built in the 1960's, backed up to The National Golf Club on Desert Inn Road in Las Vegas, NV. They loved spending their mornings and evenings in the Las Vegas sunshine away from the frozen tundra of Minnesota, where they had met in their younger years.

Dr. Mears, or Doc, as he was known to his step-daughters, owned the Chaparral Pet Clinic on Desert Inn Road, just a short two mile commute from his home. He used to travel many miles when he was a country veterinarian in Southern Minnesota covering three counties. "There's no snow to contend with," he'd say, telling others about his Minnesota practice compared to his Las Vegas practice. "I don't have to strip down to my waist in freezing temperatures to pull a calf. Now, I just have to get up in the middle of the night and work on cats or dogs," he explained. Together, they built the business from the ground up turning it into a successful practice.

The backyard at Seneca Drive created a sanctuary for the two of them. The swimming pool, surrounded by swaying palm trees, and the cool grass of the golf course, provided an oasis they only imagined in their dreams. Many happy leisurely hours were spent on the patio. Breakfast coffee sipped near the cool water was enhanced by the lush green view of the golf course. Sunrise Mountain's colors vividly changed in the background as the sun crossed the sky. Watching the golfers and their golf carts often provided a wave or a shout, "Hello". After dinner, they marveled at the changing colors of the sky and the beautiful cloud formations the desert provided while they lounged in their beautiful pool. Both of them floating on their own rafts, sometimes even gazing at the stars. Together, they adored their life on Seneca Drive.

Living next door to the golf course was Mom's delight. Known as the golf club to the stars, many famous people would pass by her yard, situated on the ninth hole. She loved working in her yard, watching the celebrities pass by. Several of them would stop and talk to her. "Tiger Woods brought his young son through the course one day," she said, "Won't it be fun to see what he accomplishes in the future," she said She enjoyed a chat with Sammy Davis, Jr.; and during the early years, she eagerly watched Arnold Palmer pass through during tournaments.

As the years passed, Mom developed a rose garden to suit a gardener's fancy. She felt a tremendous sense of pride each time she stepped into her backyard. She loved getting up at 5:00 in the morning, sitting out on her patio, sipping her coffee in the cool of the day waiting for the paper to arrive. Her twenty three rose bushes were her pride and joy, and she pruned and fussed over every single bush as if it were one of her own babies. Spurred on with the many kudos thrown her way by the local golfers, Mom loved tending to her roses, and chatting with the golfers through the ornamental wrought iron fence. "You have the prettiest yard of anyone living along the golf course," one gentleman told her.

"Why thank you!" she said, "You made my day!" The yard work seemed to fill her soul. Whether it was pruning, weeding, or mowing, she was in her glory. Cleaning her pool also made her smile. Her back yard was her oasis, and she was glad others were enjoying it, too.

Inside the house, consisting of two master bedroom suites, Mom would dust and clean to her heart's content, earning her the title of "Mrs. Clean" from her children. "I've painted the inside and the outside of this old house five times over the past forty years," she boasted. Her countless hours of decorating and re-decorating every nook and cranny were apparent the moment you stepped inside. Every wall was ensconced in elaborate decorations. Her baby grand piano was the first thing to catch your eye, and then you saw the enormous burlwood china cabinet, and dining room table which matched the burlwood of the piano. Gold glittered from every corner. Her bell collection and clown collection were spectacular works of art; and each item came with its own story. Mom was the queen of her castle; and she loved spending hours caring for it.

Once she finished her morning routine, she would shower, eat lunch and go to Chaparral Pet Clinic, where she was the office manager and bookkeeper. She ran a tight ship, often scurrying to the back section to check on a technician or client, while maintaining an upper hand on what was happening in the front office. She knew every client as well as every inch of the clinic she and Dr. Mears had built together. When they first opened the clinic, she would often serve as his emergency technician for late night emergency calls or operations. Morning and night, Mom was on the go. "I think she runs on coffee and cigarettes," I used to joke.

Before building the clinic, Mom earned extra money playing her violin in the Sands Hotel orchestra for Wayne Newton's shows. Making friends there, she loved the comraderie and excitement of playing two shows a night, but arriving home at 2:00 in the morning was difficult. "It took me so long to unwind after those performances, I often didn't get to sleep until 3:00," she said. "Then I would get up at 6:00 to make sure Bill and Lann were up for work and school. It was a grueling schedule before we got the clinic up and running."

When Bill passed away in 1994, Mom's life changed drastically. She no longer went to the clinic. It was sold to a younger veterinarian, and she threw herself into other hobbies. She put together twelve individual doll houses, furnishing them with different themes. "My favorite is this three story one," she said. "I like to call it the Rich-Bitch house!" she joked. "It even has a baby grand piano," she said proudly. Then she pointed to another smaller house. "This one is fun." she said pointing to the small cabin. "I made it for my brother, Earl. I call it Earl's fishing cabin." Every detail was special to her. "I even made a little school house in honor of you," she told me. She made a house with each of her daughters in mind, taking solace in the tedious tasks of working with the tiny items; sewing tiny curtains and miniscule bedspreads, along with building some of the furniture herself. It kept her mind off the grief and sorrow she felt after losing her special partner, Bill.

Church also became a place where she found solace in new friends, and singing in the choir every Wednesday night and Sunday morning. No longer a soprano, Mom sang tenor. "Remember the song that goes, 'Daddy sang bass?'" She laughed.

"Yes, and Momma sang tenor," I sang, using the actual tune.

"Well, now I'm the Momma who sings tenor," she joked, having always sung with us throughout our growing up years. "I used to always sing tenor with you girls, but I did it an octave higher. I guess age and smoking have taken its toll on my voice." she mused. She enjoyed helping others learn their parts.

Trying to maintain a healthy lifestyle, Mom walked the neighborhood several mornings a week, mentally counting how many steps she would walk. "I need to get to ten thousand steps," she would say. Eating like a bird, she'd have a bit of cereal at breakfast, along with her coffee. At lunch she would fix a rice cake, covered with peanut butter, and she'd add a bowl of peaches for dessert. A salad and a small portion of meat would provide her with a healthy dinner. "I've got to maintain my girlish figure," she joked, "Otherwise my clothes won't fit." She was wearing a size four or a size six petite in those days.

At the age of seventy-six, Mom attended a health fair at the Convention Center. One of the booths she encountered was about smoking. A man running the smoking cessation booth asked her if she smoked. "Why, yes, I do," Mom said.

"Would you like to see what your lungs look like?" asked the young man, showing her some possible pictures as to what her lungs might look like as a smoker.

"Okay, I'm game," said Mom, knowing that all of the health magazine articles she had read suggested quitting the smoking habit. After she completed the scan, she was aghast at the tar buildup that was covering the inside of her lungs. "I can't believe it!" she said. "After fifty years of smoking, my lungs are a mass of black tar."

Mom quit cold turkey! "That picture of my lungs made me immediately quit," she told me, describing her experience at the convention center. "It certainly wasn't easy," she said.

"How did you do it?" I asked, thinking about all of the cigarette and coffee breaks she used to take throughout her day.

"I had to change a lot of my habits and routines to get that cigarette out of my hands." she explained. "I had to hold a pen in my cigarette hand for months, but I was determined to quit. Every time I wanted a cigarette, I put a pen in my hands and I'd think about that picture of my lungs."

"Good for you!" I said, "I'm sure glad you were able to do that! I know it couldn't have been easy," I told her. Mom was proud of herself and her incredible accomplishment. She wanted to be healthy; and she was willing to tackle one of the most difficult things in life to get there. She quit smoking.

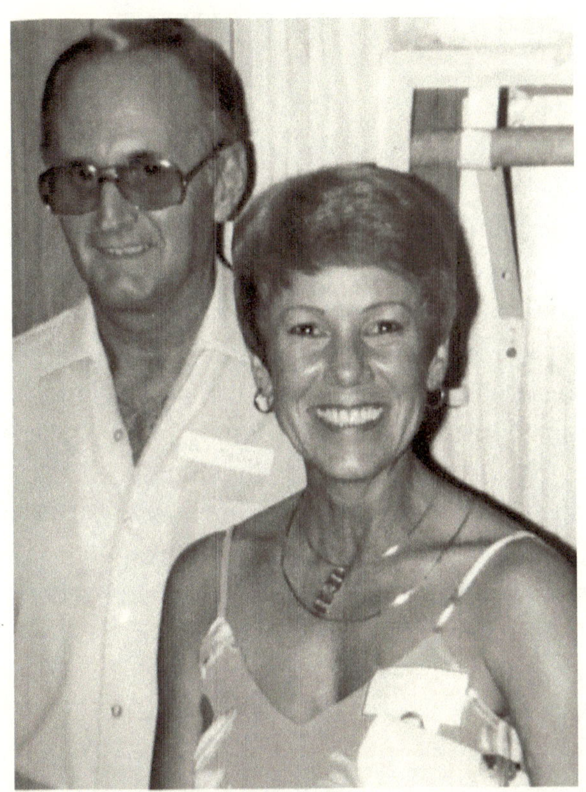

Mom and husband, Dr. Bill Mears.

CHAPTER 6

LIFE ON HER OWN

WHEN MOM REACHED the ripe old age of eighty, she had spent twenty years alone in her house, and she didn't appear to be slowing down. She continued to clean her own pool; wash the windows; climb ladders to retrieve golf balls off the flat roof of her house; and paint the house when needed. Years earlier, her husband, Bill, had aptly nicknamed her the "Energizer Bunny"! Her vitality kept her on the move, or maybe, it was the caffeine in the several cups of coffee she drank each day! However, now she knew it wasn't the nicotine! Bill would often joke about going to the airport with her. "You have to load her down with all the suitcases," he said, "otherwise, no one can keep up with her. It's like she's going to win a prize for being the first one there!"

With our visits once or twice a year, it was difficult for my sisters and I to observe Mom's gradual decline. Over the phone, she seemed quite cognizant of what she was doing, relaying daily events in detail. She ran her usual errands driving her car to the local grocery store and bank. She walked in the neighborhood every morning, and described climbing the ladder to get balls off the flat roof of her 1960's home. She seemed to be going about life as any other eighty year old woman, independently pursuing her daily routine. If she did have problems, she called Bruce, her step son who lived only a mile away. He faithfully tackled her plumbing or electrical needs. When the entire clan descended upon her for her 80th birthday, she managed to be in control of everything around her, even insisting on making meals for all twenty four of us. She reveled in all of the attention, sitting like a queen in her castle when the family gathered around her to share poems and songs in her honor. It was a joyous occasion. Little did we know she was in the beginning stages of Parkinson's.

It wasn't long after her 80th birthday party when we started noticing that Mom was slowing down. Cathy had been checking out problems with Mom's computer because it seemed to be slowing down, but what Cathy soon discovered were purchases and charges Mom had made online. Things didn't appear to be copesetic, and Cathy spent hours working on the computer, calling various companies, correcting charges, and getting money returned. Frustrated, Cathy confronted Mom, "How could you let this happen?" she yelled, choking back tears. "You've paid for two car warranties, and you're paying for things you don't even need. It makes me so mad to see how much money you've wasted!" Finally the dam broke and Cathy burst into tears, running into her bedroom, too upset to speak.

Mom sat stoically at the table, staring off in the distance; and then she looked over at me and asked, "Why is it always about money with her?"

"She's always had to be so frugal," I said. "Money is very important to her."

"I just don't understand why she gets so upset with the financial stuff," Mom said.

"Well, we're both concerned about the computer," I told her. "We don't want anyone taking advantage of you. We don't want you to get scammed on your computer." I tried to explain.

Cathy walked back into the room, "I'm sorry I yelled at you," she said. "It's just that it's so important to me that people are not taking advantage of you. There are a lot of bad people out there."

Mom was an accomplished bookkeeper; and had maintained the Chaparral Pet Clinic's records for years as well as her own household expenses. She kept them separate from the Family's Trust Fund expenses. Everyone felt she was capable of continuing this task. We just thought it was the computer that had created Mom's problems. "It's easy to accidentally push the wrong computer key and get into something a little fishy," I said, trying to impress upon Mom that she should not seek out anything new on the internet.

"Please don't click any buttons or accept any offers." Cathy said, nodding her head in agreement with me. "Just stick with emailing your friends and sharing jokes. Don't do any shopping," Cathy warned, hoping Mom wouldn't do too much damage.

When Cathy and I left Las Vegas that summer, we both felt that Mom would be perfectly capable of handling what was thrown her way. She always had, but we were wrong!

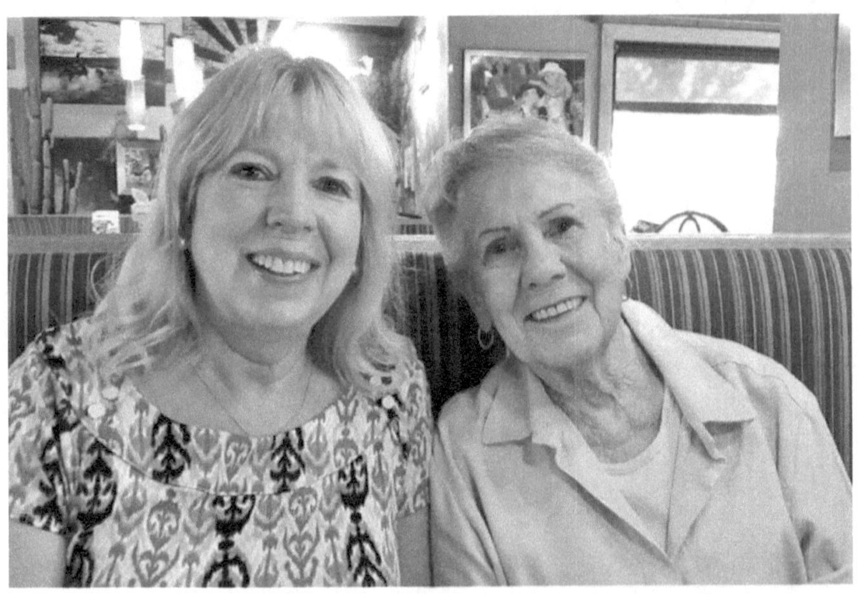

Mom with daughter, Cathy Peterson, at Applebees.

CHAPTER 7

UNRECOGNIZED SYMPTOMS

LIFE WAS SLOWLY changing. Cathy and I recognized symptoms at Mom's eighty second birthday, but we didn't realize they were symptoms for Parkinson's. The three of us headed to Wal-Mart one afternoon. Mom wanted me to drive her car. That was a change. In the past Mom had confidently maneuvered around the back roads of Las Vegas, skillfully driving us wherever we wanted to go. Now she handed me the keys and said, "Why don't you drive." It was a statement rather than a question.

It was August in Las Vegas, and the afternoon temperatures were already cooking the pavement. I was not used to the blistering heat. As I parked the car, I noticed Mom was struggling to get out of the passenger seat, so I hurried around to her side of the car, and opened the door for her. The Las Vegas heat felt like a blast furnace, and the tarmac was radiating a temperature hot enough to fry eggs. Cathy took off quickly, strutting toward the front door of the store, wanting to escape the scorching heat. I walked beside Mom who was now shuffling along at a snail's pace.

"You're embarrassed to walk with me," Mom lamented as she slowly inched along the backside of the other parked cars. "You don't like being seen with me, do you?"

"Why would you say that?" I asked continuing to match Mom's gait. "I'm right here with you." I said. "Why would I be embarrassed?" Her question took me by surprise.

"Well, Cathy doesn't want to be seen with me! Look at how far ahead she is. She's way up there," Mom said, motioning her hand in the direction where Cathy was swiftly walking, at least six car lengths ahead of us in the parking lot. "I guess I'm too slow," Mom lamented.

I chuckled. "I wonder where she learned to walk that fast?" I asked Mom. "It seems like we used to have to be speedwalkers to keep up with you! Besides, it's hotter than Hades out here, Cathy's just trying to get out of the heat. She's not used to these temperatures," I said, defending Cathy's hurried pace.

"Well, it's these shoes," Mom complained, trying to explain away her snail-paced shuffle. "It's hard to keep them on."

"Yeah," I said, "those slip-ons are difficult to walk in. I don't know how you even keep them on in the first place. They look uncomfortable."

"Well, my feet hurt," she admitted. "I feel like I'm walking on marbles, but I had to wear my green shoes because they match my outfit."

"That's true," I laughed again, "We can't have you wearing ugly shoes to Walmart now, can we?" Secretly, I was hoping I could get Mom to use one of those riding carts once we got inside the store.

Finally, shuffling through the large doors, the cool air hit us, and I said in my best English accent, "Maybe you would like to use one of these fine riding carts, Madam," I teased, hoping Mom would want to feel like a queen riding through the store. "That way, you don't have to deal with your sore feet, Mum," I joked.

"Absolutely not," Mom sneered, "I'm not using that contraption!" She waved me off and said, "I think I'll sit right here, and take a load off my feet." She immediately plunked herself down on the bench near the front door.

In the past, Mom would have led the way out in front of both of us. She was Speedy Gonzalez in a shopping mall, airport or casino; and it became an exercise in stamina for us to keep up with her. Whether we were in Safeway or Nordstroms, she was always the leader of the pack! Now, Mom was like a turtle: slothlike in her manner, shuffling her feet, inching her way one slow step at a time. And on top of that, she was admitting she was in pain. That never happened. I silently thought to myself, "It must be hell to grow old!" It never crossed my mind that something else was going on.

I began to pay attention to other elderly people, and soon discovered most of them were not doing the eighty-year old shuffle like Mom. Sure, I'd see an old man here or there, but I didn't see any women shuffling in the same manner. In fact, many of the women at Mom's retirement home were showing up for exercise classes and dance sessions. None of those people who were ambulatory were doing the eighty-year old shuffle. "This isn't part of growing old," I thought to myself. "Maybe we should get this checked out." However, life went on. Living in Washington state, my thoughts quickly turned to "Out of sight, out of mind." I didn't realize just how concerned I should have been. I've since learned small changes in the elderly should be checked out.

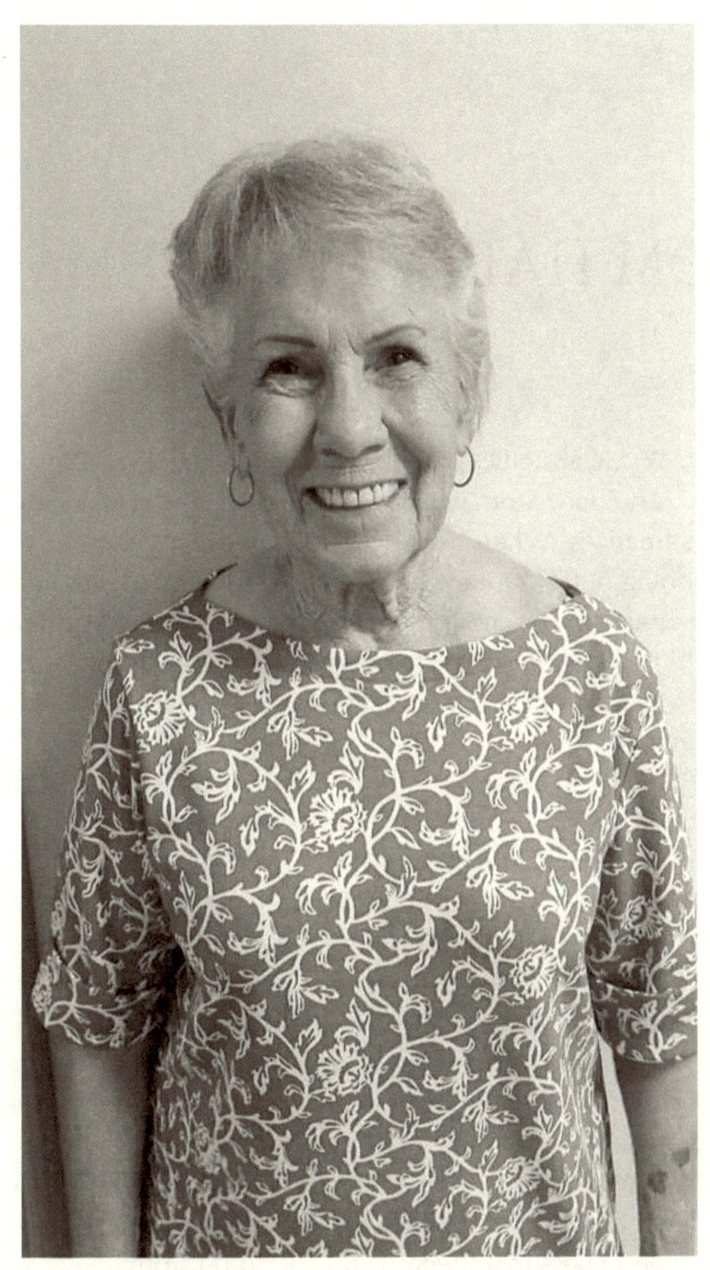

Mom before her Parkinson's diagnosis.

CHAPTER 8

MOM HAD A PROBLEM

SINCE MY HUSBAND, David, and I were the Executors for the Family Trust Fund, Mom wanted to be transparent with us about the family's finances. When her fiduciary called, notifying her that she was running out of money, he explained to her that she needed to sell her house to put more money into her fund. It was no surprise to David and I when Mom called saying, "The guy from Ameriprize called; and said that I need to sell my house because I'm running out of money."

"What should we do?" I asked David after explaining the conversation I had just experienced with Mom.

With much wisdom, David explained, "We shouldn't do anything. We can't tell your mother what to do. This is her problem and she needs to solve it herself." At first I felt as if he were being very coldhearted, but David went on to explain, "If you tell her what to do, she will be angry with you. Just be honest with her. It's her problem, and she needs to solve it. That way, she can't be mad at either one of us; and she'll more easily be able to accept the consequences."

I took the bull by the horns, calling Mom back, I said, "You definitely have a problem. If your fiduciary says you need to sell the house, then I guess that's what you need to do. You'll have to figure this out."

Five years prior to this phone call, I saw the house next door selling for $650,000. I suggested then that Mom put her house up for sale. "Look at the profit you could make if you sold your house now," I had said. "You could move into something smaller, and not have to take care of this yard and pool!" I had been excited telling her, "If you sold your house now, you could have six hundred thousand dollars in your bank account!"

Mom was having none of it. "This is the house Bill and I decided to die in. He died here, and I'm going to die here," she stated sternly. "I don't want to sell this house and I definitely don't want to move anywhere else!" She was adamant. She wasn't going to sell her house. Now, five years later, she was running out of money and her fiduciary was telling her she must sell her beloved castle. It wasn't me telling her to sell her house. David was right. She wouldn't have listened to me, even though she was running out of money, there was no way the family was going to be able to tell her what to do. She had to make the decision herself.

That is exactly what she did. Mom had been making her own decisions for twenty five years; and she would take care of this problem herself. Luckily, there was a family trust set up with a Last Testament and Will in place, so all she had to do was contact a real estate agent, list her house, and begin the process of looking for another place to live.

An acquaintance from her church lived in The Echelon Senior Living Facility, a community near her home. So one Sunday afternoon, she decided to drive the two miles up the road to visit the facility. She immediately called me and said, "I've found a wonderful retirement home, and it's close by."

"Fabulous," I said. "I'll be in Las Vegas soon, so you can show it to me when I get there. How's the sale of your house going?"

"I've shown it a few times," she said, "but it is going a little slower than I'd like." Admitting that she had become frustrated, and took the house off the market. I was shocked. She definitely needed to sell her house, but now I wondered how that was going to happen.

"Do you need a new agent?" I asked.

"No, it'll all work out," she said, and all I could do was sit back and wait. Low and behold, she put the house back on the market, and a person who had seen her house earlier, contacted the agent and said he wanted to see the house again. He ended up purchasing the house for $325,000. It wasn't the previous value of $650,000 five years ago, but at least she was going to make some money on the property. It was under contract.

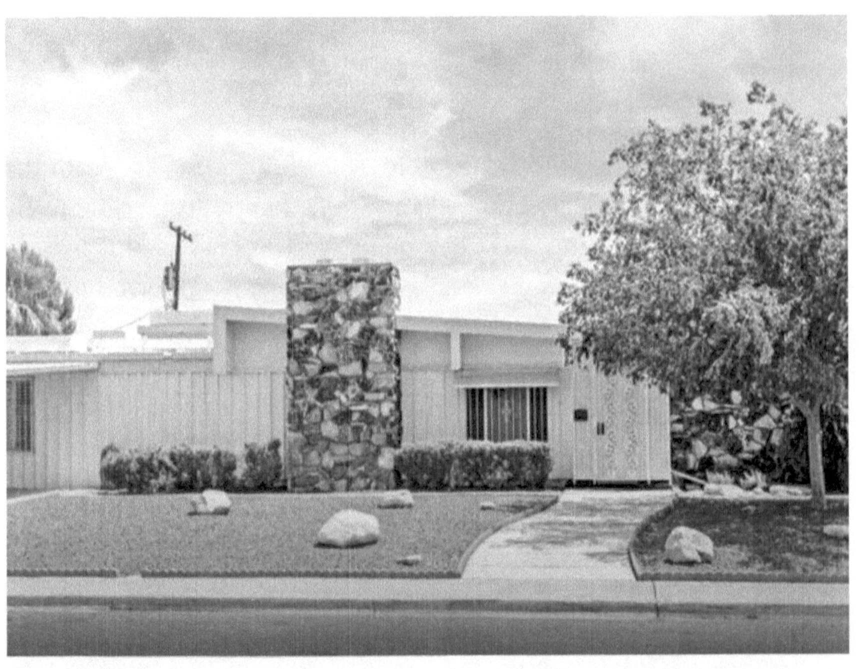

3398 Seneca Drive on National Golf Course, Las Vegas, NV.

CHAPTER 9

THE FIRST DOWNSIZING

IN 2017, HER home sold for a mere $325,000, a far cry from the $650,000 she could have gotten, but I was happy to be able to fly down to Las Vegas and help her begin the process of downsizing from her thirty-two hundred square foot home to her twelve hundred square foot retirement apartment.

Over the phone, Mom had described The Echelon apartment. "It has granite countertops and beautiful dark wood cabinets in the bathrooms and kitchen," she explained. "It also has brand new carpeting, along with a washer and dryer in its own laundry room. There is a second bedroom I can use as a sewing room and guest room." Her enthusiasm was palpable as she described the unit over the phone. Both Cathy and I were anxious to see the new place Mom had chosen.

When Cathy and I arrived in Las Vegas, Mom was excited to show us her new retirement facility. "Maybe, we should look at a couple of other places to compare what amenities they each have," I suggested, having just gone through this process with David's mother in Washington. Mom agreed to look, but after viewing one other place, she was exhausted. Getting in and out of the car was difficult for her, and walking around the facilities was even more challenging.

Much to our chagrin, when we went to look at The Echelon, the countertops were not granite, but instead covered with a thin vinyl laminate made to imitate granite. The dark wood cabinets were old cabinets recently spray painted with a black lacquer paint, still sticky to the touch, and the carpeting was not new. The previous tenant had recently passed away, so the carpeting had been cleaned. The patio was so tiny, Mom's beautiful patio furniture would not fit, but it had room for many of her plants. The downfall was that Mom would have to walk a very long distance to the dining hall. In her defense, Mom had chosen this unit, and we kept our mouths shut about its inadequacies, praising her for a marvelous decision.

Cathy and I decided to scout out two other places without Mom, and after comparing those two units, we were convinced Mom had made the right decision. Sharing a washer and dryer was not an option as it would be too far for Mom to carry her laundry, and we liked having the two bedroom unit. "We'll have our own guest room when we come to visit," said Cathy, after looking at both of the other units.

"The dining hall in the Echelon is far more cheerful, too" I said. So it was decided. We immediately made an appointment to secure the apartment at The Echelon before it was scooped up by someone else.

"She's certainly seeing things from a different perspective," Cathy said, when we were alone at Mom's house.

"Yes, even though she's had cataract surgery, I don't think she's seeing the same things we are," I said, "but she is so proud of this place, we need to keep our thoughts to ourselves." We didn't want to disappoint her. She would be devastated if she had any inkling we thought she had made a mistake.

The downsizing process began with Mom choosing pieces of furniture she wanted to take to her new home. Cathy and I made suggestions, providing our expertise on which pieces would look good in specific spaces in her new apartment. "The sofa can fit along this wall," said Cathy as we once again toured the apartment.

"Yes, and the desk with the computer can go against this bay window so she can look out at the patio," I said. Once the large items were chosen, the enormous task of getting rid of a lifetime of stuff began. Cathy, coming from Minnesota, suggested a yard sale, but Mom and I were more realistic.

"It's just too much work," said Mom, sighing with disdain.

"It's just too hot for me to stand outside for any amount of time in this Las Vegas heat," I whined. "We need to hire someone to do an estate sale," I told them. "I'll call some different places in the morning."

The next day we got in the car and drove to a Second Hand Store in Las Vegas, where we met an older gentleman who was willing to do Mom's Estate Sale. We knew a lot of work lay ahead of us, but we were pleased to be able to find someone to help us with the sale. Many of the agencies I contacted wouldn't do an estate sale where most of the large pieces were being removed from the home, even though Mom was still leaving an entire household of furniture. She was leaving a living room set, complete den, dining room table and enormous hutch, along with a baby grand piano and lots of curio cabinets.

We felt lucky Mom was still physically and mentally capable of sorting through her clothes and shoes. She was able to decide which things went to Goodwill type stores, like Safe Nest, a place which helps homeless women dress for success at job interviews, or Habitat for Humanity. Mom's petite size 4-6 clothing and size 5 shoes were not going to help many women, but she had good intentions. Sorting through her shoes, I encouraged her to give up more, but Mom said, "I need all of these different colors for my different outfits! And don't forget my winter boots. It's going to be cold walking those outside corridors to the dining hall in the winter." Mom was planning ahead and we were both proud of her decisions.

Slowly, but surely, with Mom's positive attitude, she was able to sort through her huge master closet and bathroom. Another day she sorted through her kitchen. We anticipated she was keeping more than she needed since she was provided three meals a day, but we didn't want to thwart her in the middle of the process. She managed to downsize two more bathrooms and several storage areas in her large home, but we soon realized the Energizer Bunny was slowing down. She was no longer able to heft the heavy boxes into the car or skedaddle quickly through the house. One wrong move and she could easily tumble over. We were now witnessing her lack of stability and stamina.

Cathy and I took over the task of loading up Mom's car to make several short trips over to the apartment. I hired a moving company to load the larger household items, and move them to her new apartment. Once everything was loaded, we drove over to Mom's new apartment. We had the movers place Mom's loveseat and sofa in their positions and then we placed Mom into her loveseat and explained, "You are the supervisor. Just relax. You get to tell the movers where to put the big stuff." We immediately went to work putting things into their places, while Mom gave instructions to the movers. We were moved door to door in a matter of three hours!

When the Estate Sale was all said and done, Mom's beautiful furniture didn't bring in the amount she had hoped for. The enormous burlwood dining room table that seated ten with its matching six foot long hutch, brought in pennies to the dollar, a fraction of what it was worth. The same thing happened to the matching burlwood baby grand piano. It was a sad day when Mom said goodbye to her castle at 3398 Seneca Drive. She had lived there for forty one years, and it was filled with thousands of memories, but she knew it was something she had to do. Instead of holding a grudge against David and I, she was grateful for the help we provided.

Once settled into her new apartment, Mom put a smile on her face and maintained a positive attitude, probably because she had two of her daughters with her. Lann was unable to join us, but we kept her abreast of what was happening. We knew the downside to Mom's new residence was going to be the distance that lay between her apartment and the dining hall. She was living in the farthest unit away from the dining hall; having to walk literally a quarter of a mile uphill to the dining hall to get her meals, and then walk all that way downhill back to her apartment. Mom looked at this downside with a positive spin, "I'll certainly get my exercise for the day walking to get dinner every night," she said. "It's one way to get my steps in," she laughed. She had stopped smoking twenty years earlier, and was into living a more healthy lifestyle. She looked at her long walk to the dining hall as a plus! Cathy and I were apprehensive.

Mom was paying for three square meals a day, but she decided she could fix her own coffee and cereal in the morning, and dish up her own serving of peaches and rice cake with peanut butter for lunch. She would only have to do the long walk to the dining hall for dinner. Every afternoon at 4:00, she would shuffle to the dining room for her evening meal at 4:30. If she didn't show up, the staff assured us that someone would check on her. I trusted them. The next day, Mom gave us a list of groceries to buy, and Cathy and I went shopping. We stocked up on her favorite brands of coffee; cereal, toilet paper, laundry detergent, peanut butter, peaches and rice cakes, along with her evening brandy and wine! We did not want her driving to the grocery store alone.

"Please don't drive," I said to her. "Your reaction time isn't what it used to be. If you need anything, Bruce is right up the road." Mom nodded. I had to have faith that she wouldn't be a disobedient teenager!

With Mom settled into her new domain, Cathy and I headed back to our respective homes, Minnesota and Washington, content that Mom seemed happy, and we had done the right thing. However, I was still concerned about my Mom's gait. I had secretly videotaped her walking from the car to her apartment to show David what was going on. I had gotten her a cane to help steady her tippy gate, but I had an inkling something wasn't right. I kept wondering, "Is this normal?"

After looking at my short video, David said, "That's not normal. Look at my mother," he said, "she's ten years older than you mother, and she doesn't walk like that." I began to compare every elderly person I saw to my mother. Very few were walking like Mom. When I returned to visit Mom in October, I watched the other residents who came into the dining hall. There was only one other resident that shuffled.

When I returned a few weeks later in November, I explained to Mom, "I think we need to make a doctor's appointment. You're having trouble walking, and I'm worried about you." She agreed. She, too, knew something was wrong, but didn't want to admit it. Much to my dismay, the only appointment I could get was in December. "I'll just get to spend Christmas with you in Las Vegas," I explained, trying to exude excitement in my voice.

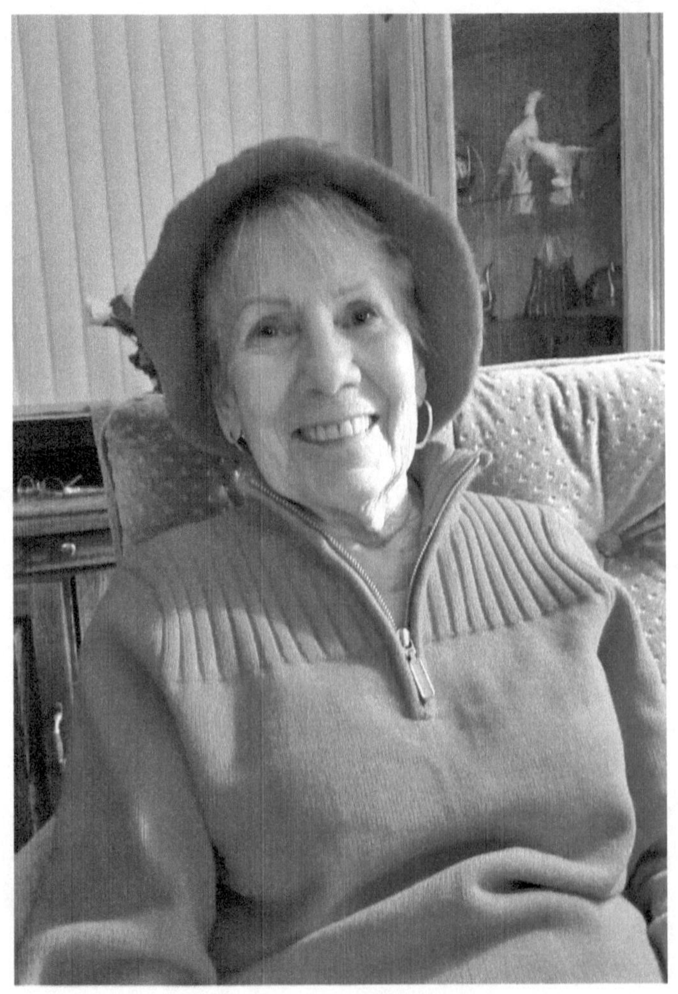

Mom, Christmas 2017 at The Eschelon in Las Vegas, NV.

CHAPTER 10

THE CHRISTMAS PRESENT

LANN, MY SISTER who lives in San Francisco, was still working, and unable to visit as often as I was. She asked me what I thought Mom could use for Christmas. She wanted to provide something useful. When I described Mom's shuffling and unsteady gait, Lann suggested getting a walker as a Christmas gift for her. "I'm sure that will help her on her long treks to the dining room," I said.

Returning to Las Vegas in December, I discovered Mom was struggling tremendously on her long journey to get her evening meals. Lann had ordered a red walker, and Cathy provided a beautiful cardinal applique to go on the bag attached to the walker. She also gave Mom a red vest emblazoned with a cardinal, Mom's favorite bird. I gave Mom a red hat and gloves to help keep her warm on her long walk across the courtyard. The walker seemed like the perfect Christmas present, and when it arrived we marveled at its shiny red frame. "It's perfect," I said. "It has a seat, so if you get tired while going across the courtyard, you can stop and rest." At the time, none of us realized walkers need to be sized for the patient. We were just impressed with the shiny red frame, the black pouch and seat. How naive we were!

One evening, after her long walk back to her apartment alone, Mom maneuvered the walker over the threshold and into her apartment and promptly fell over backwards. The enormous shiny, red walker fell on top of her as she keeled over. The large metal contraption forced her tiny frail body against the wall, pinning her to the floor. She looked like a bird caught in a large metal cage. It was only due to her sheer determination that she managed to wriggle her body out from under the king-sized walker. Once freed from the metal bars, she hobbled to the bathroom to get bandages and gauze to care for her bleeding wounds. She had scraped both shins and arms and blood had been splattered everywhere. Once her wounds were taken care of, she proceeded to clean up the blood. It seemed to be splattered on the floor and the wall. From that point on, Mom wanted nothing more to do with her shiny new walker. She would rely on her cane to get to dinner.

When we finally were able to visit Mom's general practitioner in December, her doctor said, "I'm going to send you to a specialist in Henderson. Can you get there?" she asked.

"Yes," I said. "How soon can we get an appointment?"

"He's a neurologist," said Mom's doctor, "and he will be able to help you better understand what is happening with your Mom's gait. Let me call and make an appointment for you. You'll get in more quickly if I make the appointment for you," she explained. Unfortunately, she wasn't able to obtain an appointment until January. I looked at Mom and said, "I guess I'll be back to visit in January." Mom smiled. I would fly back to Washington, take care of business there, and then fly back to Las Vegas in a few weeks. Luckily, I had a step-brother who lived in Las Vegas, and was willing to pick me up at the airport, and take me to Mom's apartment.

In January, I insisted Mom use her walker when we went to the doctor's appointment. That's where I learned a little more about walkers. Mom's walker was much too big and heavy for her small petite frame. "You should have a much lighter frame," said Dr. German, "and tennis balls on the back instead of wheels. An aluminum walker would be much better. That way she could pick up the walker as she moves forward. It will help her to keep from falling backwards." Sadly, Mom had learned this fact the hard way. She had already fallen backwards.

It soon became apparent a walker wasn't going to be the answer to help Mom get to her evening meals, and it dawned on me that we needed a caregiver; someone who could accompany Mom on her walks to her evening meals, or as I was doing, someone who could drive her around the building to the dining hall.

Hiring a caregiver is an expensive endeavor. I began calling various in-home nursing providers, and learned that part-time shifts or even split shifts were difficult to obtain. Originally I started looking for someone to check in on Mom for two hours in the morning and two hours in the evening. I wanted someone to make sure she was up and fed in the morning, and then come back to help her get to her evening meal in the late afternoon. No agency wanted a split shift, even if I increased the evening hours. Everyone wanted a full time position, and I didn't blame them.

Mom had been such an independent individual, living alone for the past twenty-five years. I couldn't imagine her having a stranger acting as her babysitter. She liked her alone time. Plus, the cost of hiring a full time caregiver was financially prohibitive. Mom couldn't afford to cover the $4,000-$10,000 a week for a full time caregiver on top of her retirement home rent because she was only getting about $1,200 in social security, the average amount most women her age receive.

Dr. German, the neurologist, had ordered an MRI of Mom's head, so Mom and I headed to the medical facility just a short drive from her apartment. She sat nervously on the cold chairs in the waiting room. Earlier in her life, she had had an MRI, and she was dreading the clanging and banging of the machine, along with the claustrophobic feeling of being on the cold table in the constricting tube. Once her name was called, I walked with her back to the changing room and helped her disrobe and put on the flimsy hospital gown.

Once the procedure was finished, the nurse brought Mom back to the changing room where I could again help her. Mom looked exhausted. "It just drains everything out of me," she said. "It's like that big magnet just zaps me of all of my strength, and it was so hard to lay on that cold hard table for such a long time!"

"We'll go home and rest," I said. "We don't have any more appointments for a few weeks.

And rest is exactly what we did. Mom requested I drive her to the dining hall, instead of walking in the cold January winds, but she was exhausted just getting in and out of the car. Sadly, when Mom went back to see Dr. German. he was upset. The MRI office had performed the wrong MRI on Mom's head. He requested she return to have the appropriate test performed.

"No way," said Mom, "I'm not going to go through that again." I didn't blame her. The clinic had made the mistake and she wasn't about to be tortured any more. Further tests performed at Dr German's neurology clinic were even more excruciatingly painful. Mom endured one test where needles were stuck into her thighs and arms and electrical currents were sent to those muscles.

"You already know she has Akinetic Rigid Parkinson's," I said, confronting Dr. German with a strong voice. "So why are you doing more tests?" I asked, after watching the technician complete the agonizing analysis.

Dr. German replied, "It will give us a better understanding of the type of Parkinson's she has and how to treat her." I didn't understand the need for all of the testing on an eighty-four year old lady who had a degenerative disease. I didn't buy the fact that they wanted to find out how they could help her. In my mind they were just doing research. I was convinced they only wanted a baseline so they could make comparisons to later test results. At Mom's age, it didn't seem like putting her through this pain was worthwhile for her.

One day, after meeting with the manager of The Echelon, Mom looked at me and asked, "Why do you always talk as if I'm not here?"

"What do you mean?" I asked.

"You talk about me to other people as if I'm not even in the room when I'm sitting right here. You're treating me like a little kid."

"Oh, I'm sorry," I said. "I hadn't realized I was doing that. As a Mom and a teacher, I have always stepped in to help others. I think it's just my nature to help. I'm sorry," I told her, realizing I often stepped in because Mom's voice was getting quieter and quieter. "I guess I feel like they can hear my voice better than your voice," I explained.

Often people with disabilities appear incapable of taking care of their own business, especially if they have a walker or wheelchair. I felt I was helping Mom, but in actuality, I was making her feel less independent. Many of the receptionists we encountered spoke to me through the window, ignoring Mom, who was standing with a cane, or sitting right next to me in a wheelchair. I began to realize how demeaning it was for Mom to be left out of the conversation about her care. I needed to work on that aspect of caregiving!

As I left the clinic that day, it was evident we needed to provide Mom with a full time caregiver. She was physically too unstable. She was still maintaining a semblance of independence, but I didn't feel comfortable leaving her alone. I decided to stay with her through the month of January. Calling Cathy, I explained my fears. She immediately made arrangements to fly to Las Vegas and stay with Mom for the month of February. Unfortunately, we still needed someone to cover the gap between our two visits. Asking around at the Echelon, I learned one of the other residents had an aide. We approached this wonderful woman, and she volunteered to help Mom get to her evening meals. She would also make sure Mom was safely settled in her apartment after the evening meal for a minimal fee. We generously paid her, and it cost much less than if we were to hire her through an agency.

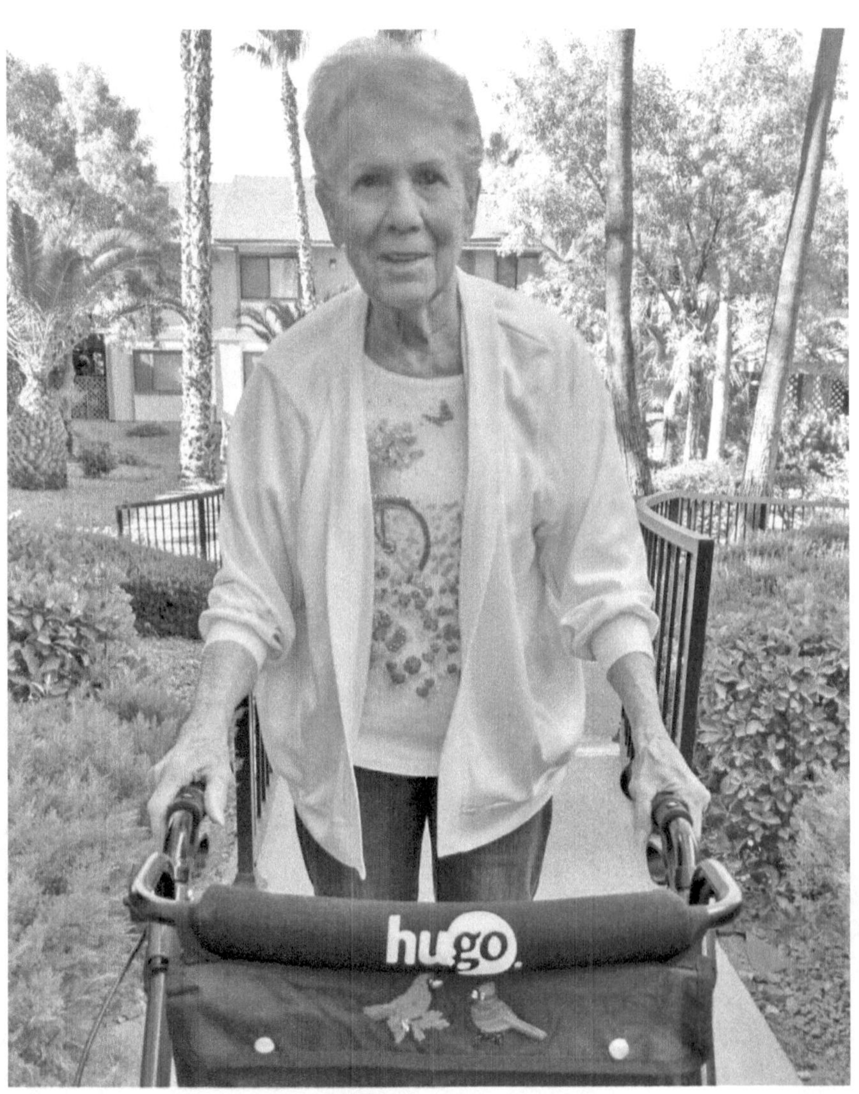

Mom with her new walker.

CHAPTER 11

THE JOURNEY BEGINS

BEFORE LEAVING LAS Vegas in January, I ordered a Life Alert Necklace. You know the kind where you press a button and say, "Help I've fallen; and I can't get up." I practiced with Mom, having her push the button a few times and asking for help. I had hoped it would give her peace of mind, knowing she could contact someone if she needed help. We installed an emergency button in her bathroom across from the toilet, next to her shower. Then we installed one near the front door where the walker had pinned her to the floor. "When you press this button, or one of the other buttons, it will contact someone." I explained. "They will call me, and we can decide what to do. It doesn't mean you have to go to the hospital," I told her. "You can just ask for help." I looked at her, and she had a confused look on her face. "Wouldn't it have been nice to have been able to push the button and have someone come and lift the walker off of you when you fell a few weeks ago?" I asked. "This little device will help you."

"But I don't want to bother anyone," Mom said, showing her hesitation to push the button.

"Oh, brother." I said, shaking my head. "Miss Independent." I chided and then added, "We're paying money for you to have this necklace, and you need to use it if you fall again," I told her. "This little necklace makes me feel better knowing you have someone to call when I can't be here."

Mom nodded, assuring me she understood.

Cathy arrived in February- two days after I had left in January. I went back to Washington state, assured in the fact that Mom had survived with our interim caregiver, and Cathy was there to continue 24/7 help. Fortunately, the lady who had previously lived in Mom's apartment had installed handicapped bars down the hall leading from the bedroom to the living room, as well as placing handicapped bars in the bathroom. I had noticed Mom was relying on those bars more than she was willing to admit. Her arms were still strong as she shuffled along the hallway, and the bars offered her a tremendous amount of confidence and support. However, one evening Mom was heading from the bathroom to her bed. There were no bars to assist her on that short journey. She fell, not quite reaching the bed, and crumpled to the floor with a thump. Cathy, hearing the noise, ran into Mom's bedroom to see if she could help, and that's when she heard Mom's feeble cry for help.

Many years earlier, Cathy had endured extensive neck surgeries after being in an elevator crash in St. Paul, Minnesota. She was not capable of lifting Mom into her bed, but somehow she managed, but not without hurting herself in the process. Now Cathy was in excruciating pain. Once Mom was settled for the night, Cathy took medication to relax her strained muscles and nerves. Both ladies were exhausted, but they had overcome their ordeal.

The next morning, they called me, both suffering maladies from the fall. As Mom explained the trauma the two of them had experienced the night before, I asked, "Why didn't you push the Life Alert Button?"

Cathy sheepishly explained, "We didn't even think of it." Embarrassed about not remembering to ask for help, she said, "We were just working so hard to get Mom into her bed that we didn't even think about the necklace."

Eventually, I explained to our volunteer caregiver, "I purchased the Life Alert Necklace for a reason. I hope you remember to use it, if you need it." I described Cathy's ordeal. I wanted her to know that

Mom had the necklace as another layer of security. The necklace gave me a sense of security, but in the long run, it is not worth anything if it isn't used.

Cathy's visit to Las Vegas got off to a rocky start, helping Mom off the floor and into her bed. She was in pain. Next Cathy took Mom to a follow up appointment with Dr. German. Thinking the doctor knew best, we had kept the appointment, not understanding that this next visit would entail more excruciating tests. When Mom and Cathy settled in the exam room, the technician began a hearing test, but this hearing test was completely different from the ones we were accustomed to. "They stuck needles into Mom's ears; and tested her hearing by sending electrical shocks into her ears," said Cathy. "I couldn't watch!"

Finally, Mom cried, "Enough! Just stop! You've already told me I have Parkinson's. I can't do this anymore. I'm done." If she could have jumped off the table, she would have run out of the room as fast as she could.

"I couldn't believe what they were doing!" said Cathy when she called me on the phone. "It seemed too painful to fathom what was happening," she added.

Mom was on the speaker phone and spoke up. "Why should I pay money to be tortured?" she asked.

"You certainly have a point," I said, feeling total empathy for my mother having had to endure such an excruciating test.

"I feel like a guinea pig," she said.

"Well, I think we'll just skip any more appointments at Dr. German's office," I told her, "We already know you have Parkinson's; and we already know there is no medication that will help you."

Mom sighed, "Thank you." There would be no more testing.

After Cathy's visit to Dr. German's office ended with a negative taste in her mouth, she and Mom returned home to spend their days chatting and sorting through the items that had been rather quickly stashed into cupboards and closets during Mom's hasty move. Mom was enjoying her new recliner; which Cathy hadn't seen before.

One day Cathy asked Mom, "Why aren't you using the electric lift on your chair?"

"I have two reasons," Mom said with a smile, "I don't like waiting for it to raise me up; it seems like it takes forever, and besides," she continued, "I want to keep my arms and legs working as long as possible, so I'm trying to keep up my strength."

Mom was right. When I was there in January, I learned that one of the most important things Parkinson's patients can do for themselves is to continue to exercise. Aerobic exercises are paramount to keeping the muscles strong. They can also provide a fun social activity, such as dancing, Tai chi, or yoga strength training. Cross body activities also keep the brain functioning at its maximum. I downloaded some Youtube videos and tried to help Mom work on cross body movements. She became very frustrated with simple clapping and patting, and lifting alternate legs. Even the simplest of cross body pats and claps were frustrating for her brain, and she refused to work with me. I think she thought it was baby stuff. She often said, "I don't want to do any of that Kindergarten stuff." Instead, she had been pulling herself up by using the coffee table to lift herself up out of the recliner, thinking she was keeping her arms strong. She did have strong arms and legs, and moving around her apartment independently was paramount for her mental attitude.

Her apartment was small enough that she didn't really need much help. She was still able to get out of bed by herself in the morning; go to the bathroom on her own; brush her own teeth, and walk down the hall to the front door. Using the handicapped bars to insure her safety, she tottered along the hallway. As she rounded the corner past the laundry room, she would use the door handles and the credenza to manage getting safely to the front door. There, she would unlock the door, reach around to the front of the large heavy wrought iron screen door, and grab her morning newspaper. The handicap bars and her cane provided her with the sense of security she needed to stay independent.

Shuffling a few steps, Mom would go into the kitchen where she made her own coffee, and got her breakfast ready. Standing at the sink, she lifted the small cereal bowl out of the strainer, and reached into the cupboard for the cereal. I had previously placed the cereal into small ziplock baggies, making it more convenient for her to get her own breakfast rather than lifting a heavy cereal box. Her usual breakfast consisted of a small bowl of cereal with a little milk, along with her coffee. Turning and shuffling just a few steps, she was able to set the bowl on the kitchen table. Maneuvering back to the sink, she poured herself just a half cup of coffee to avoid spillage. Shuffling back to the table, she smiled to herself. Everything in her new apartment was so compact. She could still enjoy the same routine she had enjoyed all those years at Seneca Drive. She was independent and loved it.

Once Mom finished her breakfast, she washed her spoon and bowl at the kitchen sink, and set them in the strainer to dry. "I'll just use them again for lunch with my peaches," she told me when I offered to wash them for her. Pouring herself another cup of coffee, she shuffled around the table, and grabbed her newspaper to settle herself into her recliner. It was funny watching her. As she read each page, she threw the discarded pages onto the floor next to her recliner; and then she began to fold the page with the crossword puzzle. I noticed it wasn't the perfect folds she used to do as she struggled with the large piece of newspaper print; but somehow she managed to get the crossword puzzle into a position where she could read and write at the same time. Although her writing had begun to shrink to chicken scratching, she usually remembered what she had written. Her words were barely legible to me, but Mom still continued to work on solving every clue. "I need to keep my mind sharp," she said as she solved each clue, often gazing into the distance and pondering on what the answer could be.

Eventually, solving the crossword puzzles became one of the things Mom and I would do together. I would read the clues out loud, and she would think a minute, then tell me the answer. I'd write the answer onto the paper, and read another clue. Her vocabulary was phenomenal. She was used to working on three crossword puzzles a day, and her proficiency outweighed mine by a long shot. I needed to physically see the spaces and clues and how they fit together, but Mom could visualize them in her head. She was a sharp cookie, continuing to try to read everyday keeping her mind alert. I was impressed with her mental abilities. I didn't know how long this strong independence would last, but we were hopeful.

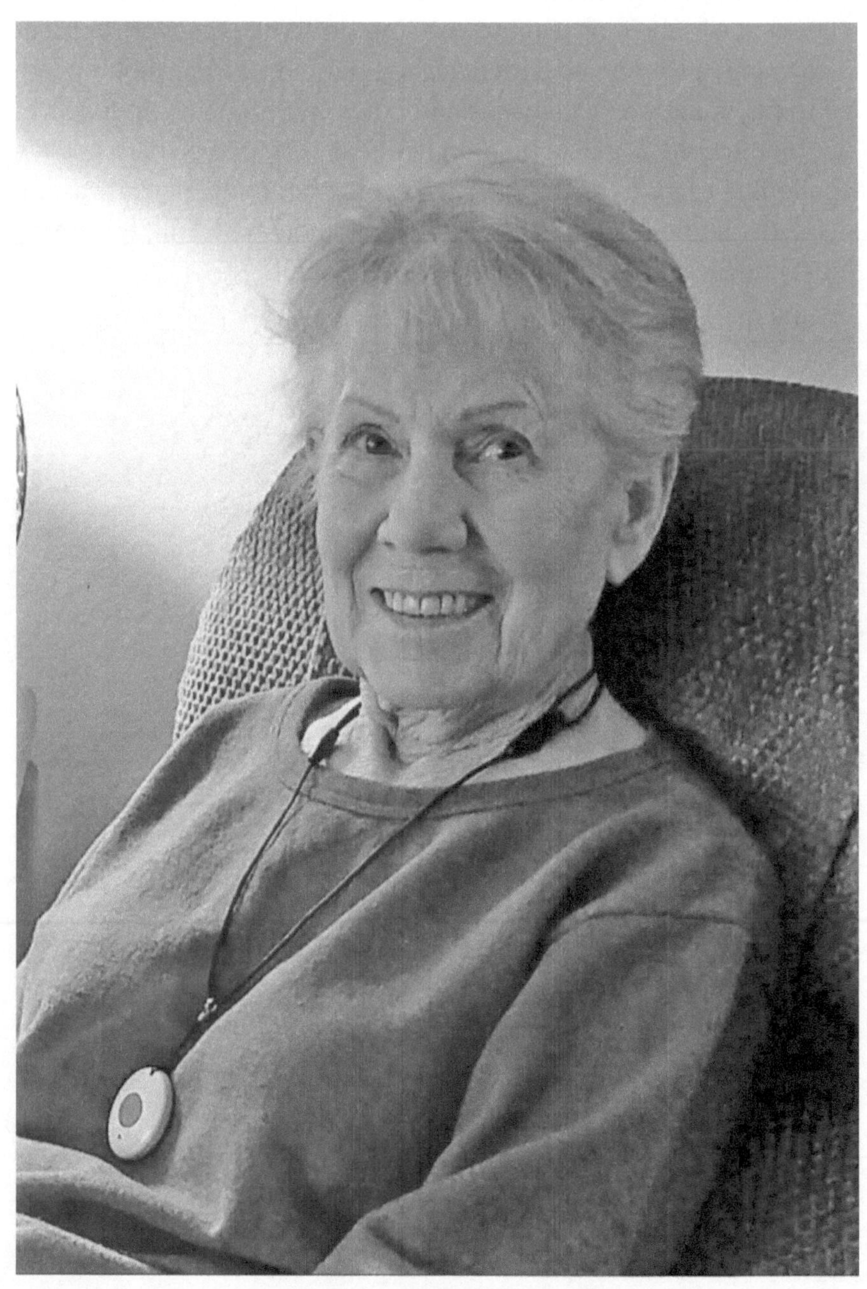

Mom with her Life Alert Necklace.

CHAPTER 12

LIFE CHANGED IN AN INSTANT

SUDDENLY, A BOUT of diarrhea changed everything. Mom's eighty year old shuffle complicated her efficiency getting to the bathroom quickly, and she was tremendously embarrassed to have Cathy help her get cleaned up. When Mom called me to tell me about the day's events; she sadly said, "I didn't make it to the bathroom. I had the worst diarrhea of my life. It was so embarrassing. It reminded me of the time when I was in first grade. I was in the old one room schoolhouse in Wells, Minnesota, and the big boys in the school were always teasing me about being the littlest kid and the slowest eater."

"How old were the boys?" I asked, having already heard Mom tell this story; but I let her go on because I wasn't sure if Cathy had heard the story.

"They were 7th and 8th graders," she told me. Her voice became soft and quivering as she remembered the incident.

"What did they do to you?" I asked her. "I can't imagine having all of those grades in a one room schoolhouse," I added, reminiscing about my own teaching days.

"Well, one day we were outside for lunch; and the teacher rang the school bell for us to come in from lunch recess," Mom explained. "When everyone was settled in their desks, the teacher looked around and discovered I wasn't at my desk. Since I was the littlest, I always sat at the littlest desk in the front of the room," Mom said. "I guess when the teacher looked up and discovered I wasn't there, she asked the other students where I was. They told her I was still outside. She went outside and called my name; and when I didn't answer, she came looking for me. I was screaming for help!"

"Oh my gosh," I gasped. "What happened to you?"

"The big boys had hung me up on a hook at the back of the out-house with the loops of my overalls. I had messed my pants; and I was so embarrassed," she said. "The teacher had to lift me down and help me get cleaned up. Ever since that awful experience, I've always been so conscientious about making it to the bathroom on time. Today was devastating;" she said, "and it wasn't just one time. I didn't make it several times; and Cathy has had to help me clean up the bathroom, the rugs, and me!"

"Oh! I'm sorry you had to go through that. Was Cathy okay helping you?" I asked, knowing Cathy was embarrassed easily.

I could tell Mom had turned to Cathy while she was still on the phone with me and said, "I'm so sorry you had to clean up that mess."

"I'm so glad Cathy was there to help you," I reassured her, "I'm sure she was happy to help."

Cathy had diligently dug in, cleaning the carpet and wiping down the bathroom; while Mom worked to clean herself up in her own bathroom. Unfortunately, they had no idea Mom had C.diff, a highly contagious digestive disease caused by the Clostridioides difficile bacteria. It is often associated with someone who has been taking antibiotics in the hospital, but that hadn't been the case for Mom. She hadn't been in the hospital or taking any antibiotics, so we attributed the C.diff to the fact that Mom hadn't been washing her hands thoroughly after using the bathroom. On top of the lack of hygiene, Mom had been using dental picks to clean her teeth. The combination of not washing her hands; and then having her hands near her mouth proved to be a deadly combination. It was a perfect setting for C.diff to colonize in her body. The transfer of bacteria from her hands into her mouth had caused the C.diff infection to become quite severe, and made watery bowels occur several times that day.

As sisters, Cathy and I had privately discussed the need to get more extensive care for Mom. We looked at various assisted living facilities online, but we were struggling to juggle our schedules so we could take turns traveling back and forth from our own homes to Las Vegas to oversee Mom's care. It was becoming apparent to us that we weren't doing the best for Mom. Although we were both retired, we both had other commitment;s and neither one of us could care for Mom full time. Mom had previously stated she did not want to live with either one of us. "You both need to live your own lives," she had said, "I don't want to be a burden." The key to making Mom happy was to have her in the nicest facility she could afford. After checking out four different facilities, we chose The Bridge, located just a few blocks from The Echelon. We explained to Mom what we were up to, and made arrangements for Nurse Ann and Director Danielle from The Bridge to visit Mom at The Echelon and interview her. Mom understood, these two ladies wanted to help us find a place where she would have more help.

Luckily, Mom was cleaned up when the two women arrived for the interview that afternoon. They completed their medical evaluation to determine the level of care Mom would need. They would also determine whether their facility would be a good fit for Mom. These two ladies graciously conducted their interview; asking Mom and Cathy several questions about her daily abilities. Then, as they were leaving, they met Cathy quietly by the front door. "Your Mom is very sick," said Danielle. "She has a serious infection, and needs to get to the hospital immediately," said Ann, her nursing skills kicking in. "We can literally smell the C.diff, which is a life-threatening diarrhea."

Unbeknownst to Cathy, diarrhea from C.diff smells very foul. She wasn't aware that when an elderly individual has three or more bouts of watery diarrhea a day, they need medical intervention to ensure they do not become dehydrated. Mom certainly wasn't drinking enough water, and probably was becoming dehydrated. Fortunately, these two ladies' medical knowledge was invaluable. They recognized the smell of C.diff, and were not afraid to alert Cathy to the impending devastation. Evidently the little apartment wreaked with the pungent odor of this nasty disease, alerting them to voice their concern, which literally saved Mom's life.

Cathy, unable to get Mom to the hospital on her own, called our brother, Bruce. He lived just blocks away; and when he arrived, they determined there was no way they could physically get Mom to the hospital on their own. It was time to push the Life Alert Button and summon an ambulance. The ambulance arrived, and Mom was transported to Desert Springs Hospital just a few blocks from her home. Since I was the contact person for the Life Alert Button, I was called, and I was thrilled to report the system worked.

As the designee on Mom's medical directive, I made arrangements to fly down to Las Vegas; happy I was able to provide Cathy some support. She was able to meet me at the airpor;t and we were both fortunate to be able to stay in the guest room at Mom's apartment. Later, when we moved Mom out of her apartment at The Echelon, Bruce was kind enough to allow us to use his two guest rooms. Living accommodations are often expensive when you don't have family in the area.

Initially, after being taken to Desert Springs Hospital in her neighborhood, Mom's insurance insisted she be transferred immediately to Mountain Ridge Hospital across town. Dr. Kumar began treatment for her C.diff infection with megadoses of antibiotics. It took a week for those strong medications to knock the C-Diff out of her body. We visited Mom every day, making the half an hour drive over to that hospital, as did many of her friends.

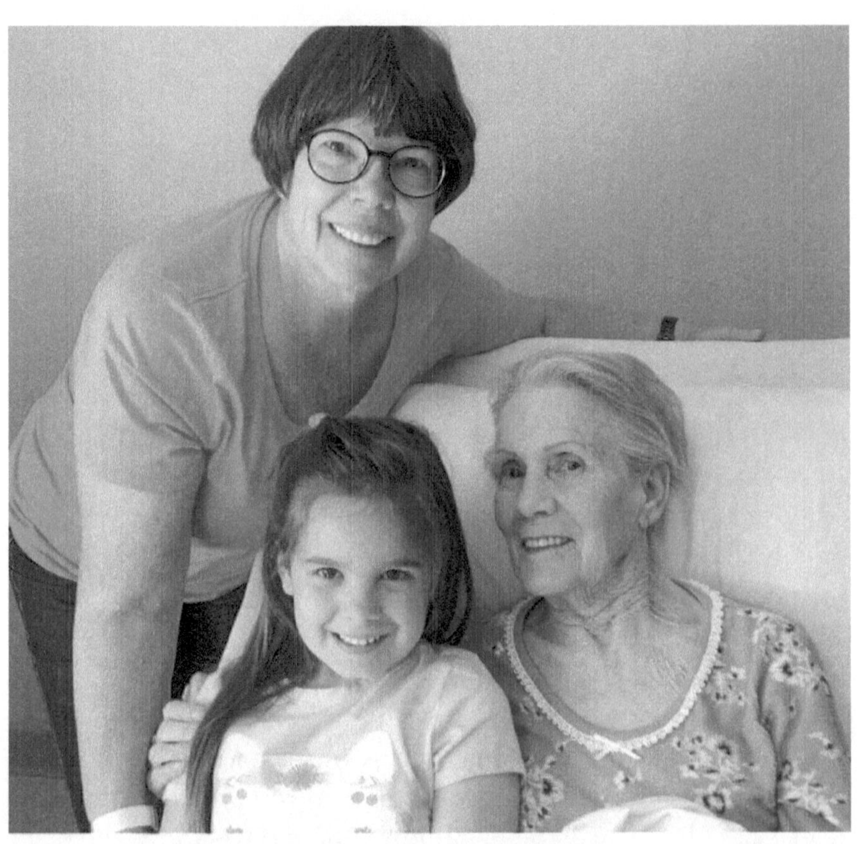

Mom with Caryn and great granddaughter, Legend,
at the Life Care Facility.

CHAPTER 13

RESEARCHING A REHAB FACILITY

WHEN MOM WAS ready to be released from the hospital, we were told we needed to choose a rehab facility for her. Our sole goal was rather selfish. We wanted to keep Mom close to her home area. Having already chosen The Bridge as her assisted living facility, we decided to choose Life Care Of Las Vegas, a sister community, located right next to The Bridge. We had already started the admission process at The Bridge, so we felt it would provide an easy transition. Plus, it was conveniently located near Bruce's home. It enabled Cathy and me to have a short commute from his house to Mom's new facility. By keeping Mom in her surrounding neighborhood, it meant Cathy and I were also familiar with the area. In hindsight, we highly recommend researching the online reviews of all the available facilities. Little did we know, the place we had chosen had very low ratings. Not only were they extremely short staffed; but the care by those staff members was inferior. If only we had read the reviews. We understand the facility is now under review by Medicare.

Having spent a week in the hospital, Mom was ready and willing to go home. It was difficult when we had to tell her she was going to a Skilled Nursing Facility for rehabilitation.

"Why am I here?" Mom asked when we met her at the Life Care Facility.

"The doctor wants you to stay here and get your strength back," I told her. She looked very pale from her ordeal at the hospital. "They have therapists who will work with you and help you get stronger," I said. The doctor wanted Mom to have physical therapy as well as occupational therapy to help her gain her strength back. They were hoping she could get back to walking independently again. Unfortunately, Mom's positive attitude took a nosedive; and she fell into a state of depression that we had not experienced since she lost her husband twenty five years earlier.

Once her husband passed away in 1994, Mom stayed very close to home. She loved her house. It was her castle, and she was the queen. The week in the hospital was enough to do her in; but now she was going to be spending a month in a rehab facility. Emaciated and frail, Mom was mortified to find out they were putting her in diapers. She refused to get dressed. She spent her days laying in her hospital gown, in her bed with a scowl on her face. Constantly calling the nurses' station for assistance using the restroom, she became highly agitated and grumpy. She refused to use the diapers they had put on her; and when the nursing assistants weren't prompt, she became perturbed. Although she couldn't yell, she was not the kind woman she had been. It was difficult watching this sophisticated woman lose her dignity. My only hope was that a physical therapist could help her gain her strength and vivaciousness back.

With daily encouragement, Mom grudgingly participated in Occupational and Physical Therapies which were provided by her insurance. Each day, one doctor or another would come to her room, cajoling her into cooperating with their antics. The first week, they worked with her in her room, coaxing her out of her bed, pushing her to stand, and helping her to maneuver her body into her wheelchair. They began a program to build her strength in hopes she would be able to get to her wheelchair and propel herself around. After a week of therapy in her room, they wheeled her down to the therapy room, where they had more equipment to help build her strength.

Unbeknownst to the therapists, Mom had a very tender spot on her tailbone. It was the beginning of a bedsore which became progressively more debilitating over time. One of the physical therapists had Mom use her arms to lift herself up and slide her bottom across a leather bench. As she did this, she continually rubbed the bedsore. The grimaces on her face should have warned the therapists of her discomfort. Too embarrassed to explain her problem, Mom just refused to participate in physical therapy.

For an entire month, the various therapists worked with Mom, trying to get her to stand without falling over, and walk with the aid of a walker. They worked at getting her to propel her own wheelchair, building up her arm strength to push her own wheels, and use her feet to inch herself forward. But sadly, Mom's frail body and depressed mental state hindered her ability to move forward. She desperately wanted to use her walker and maintain some of her independence, but her instability caused the staff to say, "We can't let you walk alone. You're too prone to fall backwards or sideways. We need two people to be with you at all times, and quite frankly, we don't have enough staff to let you use the walker outside of the therapy room."

Mom couldn't stand on her own, and she couldn't propel herself in the wheelchair. She became wheelchair bound, and was totally dependent on having someone push her. Even though they continually worked with her to gain more stability, insurance deemed it time for her to move out of the rehab center. Mom was more than ready to go!

During Mom's stay at the Life Care Facility, she had become very frustrated with the food situation. She refused to go to the dining hall, but instead had food brought to her room as if she were an invalid. When the food arrived, she couldn't cut it and she had trouble maneuvering the utensils. She'd lost so much strength during the one week stay in the hospital, she ended up eating many things with her fingers. Cathy purchased silverware specifically designed with the Parkinson's patient in mind. They were weighted, which kept the utensil and the food more stable. Mom tried them once, and then refused to be burdened with their heaviness. "These aren't going to work," she declared and we put them away.

When Mom had lived at The Echelon, she had experienced various table mates. One night, Lois, a classy woman, joined Mom and me for dinner. Lois needed to eat with her fingers. She picked through her food; and Mom thought it was disgusting to watch. To add insult to Mom's misery, Lois had two inches of polished fingernails which curved around the ends of her fingers. Mom wasn't impressed. Later that night, Mom asked me, "Did you see her long, dirty fingernails?"

"Yes," I said, "I wonder who does her manicures."

"They're filthy," Mom said as we slowly walked back to her apartment. "Those long fingernails are caked with dried food; and her fingers are all greasy. Watching her eat made me gag!"

"Well, she's doing the best she can," I said.

Now, at the Life Care Facility, this conversation played back in my mind; and it was probably playing back in Mom's memory as well. She was probably thinking about Lois and she didn't want anyone to see her eat with her fingers. I tried to be at Mom's side for lunch and dinner to assist her in cutting her food, or opening various packages, but breakfast was a different story. I couldn't get there in time for breakfast, and she was very irritated. "Can't they serve something other than those ridiculous fake scrambled eggs?" she asked. "It's impossible to keep them on my fork."

"I'll ask the cook," I said, wondering what the cook would have to say about Mom's critique.

Later in the day, I was able to head down to the kitchen where I found the head chef available to chat. Explaining Mom's dilemma as a Parkinson's patient, he replied, "Yes, those scrambled eggs tend to roll up into little balls when we stir them."

"Well, you can imagine a Parkinson's patient trying to keep those little balls on their trembling fork!" I laughed, as I demonstrated a fork held by someone with tremors. "My mother isn't impressed!" I said.

"There are lots of other choices," he said, getting out the menu to show me the options for breakfast.

"Oh my gosh!" I said. "No one has shown my mom that she has choices. They have just been bringing her the same thing every morning because we didn't know she had all of these options." I was astonished. Not one nurse in the place had asked my Mom what she would like for breakfast. It had been easier to just bring her the same thing every morning. "Meals are difficult for her," I told the chef. "Thank you so much for your help!" I said, as I left the kitchen walking back to Mom's room.

No offense to the chef, but Mom lost ten pounds while living at the Life Care Facility, partially due to her depression, and partially due to her inability to navigate the food. I was surprised they didn't have a nurse make sure she was able to eat what was placed in front of her. She barely had the energy to lift the large plastic covers off of the plates. She had eaten the same thing for lunch for the past twenty-five years and this dietary change threw her for a loop. It was difficult for her. By April 1st, when she was moved via wheelchair and ambulance to The Bridge, her eighty six pound weight made her look frail and emaciated. I knew hospice was the right decision.

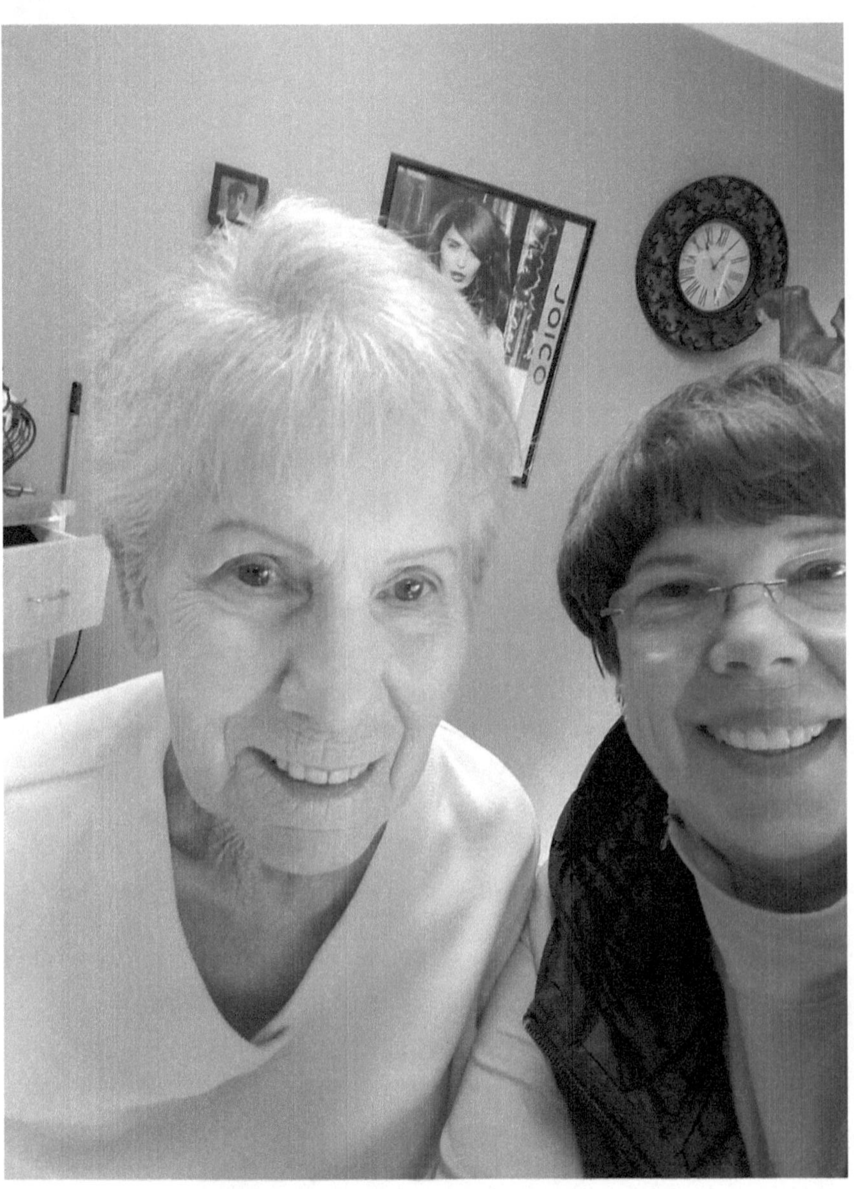

Mom and Caryn Mears made a quick trip to Mom's favorite beauty shop.

CHAPTER 14

WHO'S MANAGING YOUR MEDICARE?

EVEN THOUGH CATHY and I were eager to have Mom move into her new room at The Bridge, no one was more eager than Mom herself. However, before Mom could move into the assisted living home, there were several hoops we needed to jump through to get her there. One of the hoops was to get Mom qualified for a hospice program. Several staff members at the Life Care Facility recommended Mom change from a managed Medicare program to regular Medicare. "She'll be able to get more services under the regular Medicare program," they informed me. "Under her managed care, she has to follow their rules, and they are restricting how long she can receive rehabilitation. They're the ones that made her go to the hospital across town," they informed me.

Just like everyone else, when Mom turned sixty-five, she had signed up for Medicare. Living alone and trying to save money, she signed up for a managed Medicare program called Senior Dimensions. With this program, she paid smaller amounts for her doctor's visits and medications, not realizing they were going to limit who she could see for those doctor visits. She thought she was saving money when she chose Senior Dimensions Managed Care of Southern Nevada. They did serve her well over the years, providing low payments for doctors' visits and for medications, although they limited which doctors she could see. In the long run, it appeared to be financially the best choice at the time. Now, Senior Dimensions was limiting how long she could be in rehab and receive therapy.

"Managed care," said one of the nurses at Life Care Facility, "will not allow your Mom to stay here more than thirty days, and we both know she needs a longer rehabilitation period than that. Basically Senior Dimensions is limiting the services she can receive." She further explained, "Regular Medicare would allow her to stay as long as needed."

Although I didn't want Mom to stay in the Life Care Facility any longer than necessary, I did listen to their advice. Contacting Senior Dimensions, I made an appointment to meet with one of their counselors. On the day of my appointment, I took Mom's Medicare card, her social security card, her driver's license, and the paperwork showing me as the Power of Attorney, as well as her health care directive, indicating I was in charge of Mom's medical decisions. I was prepared with all the documentation I needed, along with her Senior Dimensions card and account number.

"I'd like to disenroll my mother from your managed care program," I said when I was finally invited into a counselor's office.

"This is highly unusual," said the woman, looking very dismayed with a frown crossing her face.

"I understand," I said, "but at this stage of my Mom's life, I feel she will get better services through the regular Medicare program. What do I need to sign?" I asked.

"These forms need to be signed in triplicate," said the counselor. "There is a copy for you, a copy for us, and one will be sent to Medicare." The counselor shook her head as she watched me sign the various papers. I tried to act confident in my decision, but deep down inside I was still second guessing myself.

As I walked out of the building, I headed to Mom's car and pondered my decision. "Am I really doing the right thing?" I asked myself when I sat down in the driver's seat. Before starting the car, I telephoned Cathy. "I just took Mom off the Senior Dimensions managed care, and now we need to get her some other kind of insurance. I guess we need a supplement to Medicare," I explained to my sister.

"I've been looking at that for myself," she said. "I can check that out from here." I was relieved to have her on board.

"I sure wish there was a manual on how to care for parents," I joked.

"Well, we didn't have one when we had our kids, so I guess we'll have to learn by trial and error with our parents, too," she laughed. "Let me start looking for a secondary insurance," she said, "and I'll get back to you." We hung up. She was back in Minnesota and could easily do a quick computer search for insurance companies while I drove back to visit Mom. Cathy later called me and said she had found an affordable secondary insurance plan for Mom, as well as a Part D plan which was necessary to help pay for Mom's medications.

"Part D stands for Drugs!" Cathy said, when she called back. "Silver Script is the name of the company. They will order the prescriptions and have them sent directly to The Bridge." She gave me the phone number and address so I could contact them with Mom's medical information. Once we had Mom enrolled in additional insurance plans, it felt like nothing had changed. Cathy was able to have the same pharmacy send Mom's prescriptions over to the nurse at The Bridge. Things were falling into place, but we had another hoop to jump through.

Although we had several meetings with the nursing staff and financial staff from The Bridge, we still needed to get Mom enrolled in a hospice program. According to staff at The Bridge, Mom's care would be enhanced if she were enrolled in a hospice program prior to her arrival.

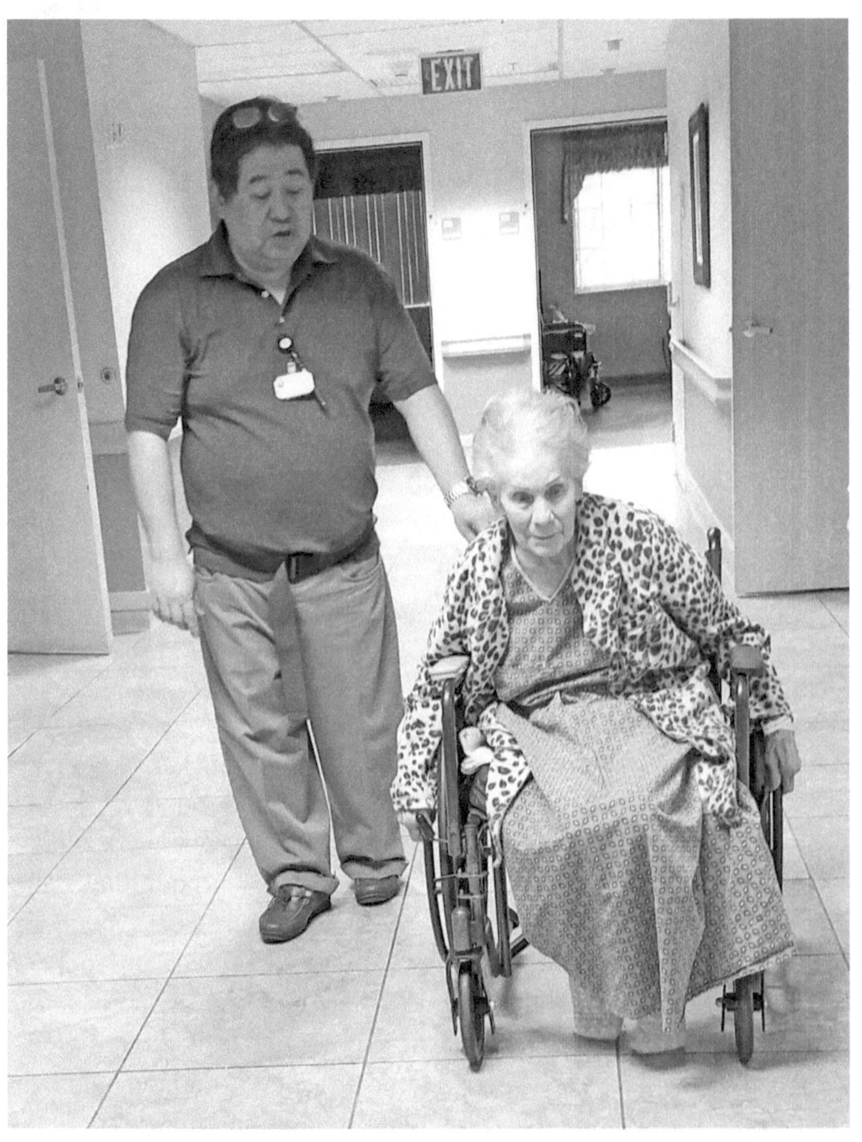

Mom is learning to move her own wheelchair at the Life Care Facility

CHAPTER 15

MOVING TO ASSISTED LIVING

WHILE MOM HAD been in rehab at the Life Care Center, Cathy, Bruce and I had worked behind the scenes to pack up Mom's belongings at The Echelon. We knew she was no longer capable of living at the senior retirement home, and we also knew once she was released from the skilled nursing facility, she needed an assisted living facility. None of us had the capability of caring for her in Las Vegas, and Mom didn't want to leave Las Vegas.

I called my daughter, Mimi, who was living in Las Vegas, and asked her husband, Rob, to join Bruce, Cathy and me as we moved Mom's possessions from The Echelon to The Bridge. What we couldn't fit into her room at The Bridge, we took to a storage unit that Cathy and I had secured the week before. With two family trucks, two cars, and five adults, we were able to take Mom's bed, dresser, and recliner, along with two chairs, and lots of boxes, over to her new room at The Bridge before she had officially arrived. Then we took the remaining bed, night stands, dresser, kitchen table and chairs, and twenty boxes over to the storage unit. We didn't know how long that storage unit would be needed, but we were glad we had it.

The entire family worked together to make Mom's room as comfortable as possible. Cathy and I wanted her to feel the same ambiance she felt in her home on Seneca Drive, so we filled her new room with her favorite possessions. "You know, in six months Mom's moved from a three thousand square foot home to a twelve hundred square foot apartment, to a four hundred square foot room," said Cathy. "She's lost a lot in a very short time."

"You're right," I said. "She's faced a tremendous amount of upheaval in her life, but this is by far the one that is going to be the most difficult for her." I said while arranging books and pictures on the bookcase shelves, "I'm glad you had the idea of getting this bookcase." I added, "It's perfect for displaying her favorite clowns and bells. That'll make her happy."

"I'm putting her violin up above this cupboard," Cathy said, standing on a step stool reaching far above her head. "She can't play it, but she needs it to stay here with her."

"Great," I replied, carrying Mom's beautiful clock over to Cathy. "Lann gave her this clock. You might as well put it up there, too, as I don't know where else to put it. She can't have it chiming in here at night."

"Thanks," said Cathy, looking around the room. "Let's put her trunk under the mirror," she said, as she stepped down from the stool, heading over to the trunk.

"Wait!" I gasped. "I want to see what's inside that trunk before we push it against the wall." We both walked over to the shiny gold foot locker sitting in the middle of the floor. Together, we bent down; and Cathy pulled the flat floral pillow off from the top. Mom had made the cushion to protect the shiny top from being scratched. Cathy laid the pillow on the bed, as I reached over to unlock the center clasp. Mom had used the footlocker at the end of her guest bed to hold the comforter when it wasn't being used. I remembered Mom showing me several keepsakes she had stored inside, and I had hoped they were still there.

As we lifted the shiny lid, we were treated to the sight of the treasures I remembered. We found the scrapbook Mom had put together from her reign as Mrs. Minnesota in 1965. I was thirteen years old then; and that huge brown scrapbook held our family's history for that one very special year. I remembered going to the airport and waving goodbye to my Mom and dad as they headed to San Diego where Mom would compete in the Mrs. America pageant. The picture in that book shows me standing next to my parents, a gawky preteen with a funky hair style and braces.

We carefully turned the fragile pages, remembering the time the local newspaper photographer visited our house and took the pictures held in the book. Those pictures were all safely tucked inside, along with our history. Mom had captured it so well, and now the book was housed in the gold foot locker, the safest place she knew.

Everything was there in that trunk, just as I had remembered it, even Mom's record album from when she played the violin at the Sands Hotel with Wayne Newton. She had playbills from her favorite Las Vegas shows and special pictures of her brother, whom she'd located when she was fifty years old. Mom was very proud of the treasures stored in that trunk, and I knew it wouldn't be the last time we looked at them.

"This scrap book is almost fifty five years old!" said Cathy, carefully closing the book and placing it back in the trunk.

"That's certainly a long time ago," I said as we closed the trunk and slid it across the floor to its new resting place.

Looking around the room, I could see Mom's photo albums neatly lined up on the shelves of her new bookcase. Nestled amongst her favorite knickknacks were her clowns and bells, pared down from her once massive collections. Her clothes hung neatly in the closet, shoes placed methodically on the floor below with her pajamas, sweater sets and lingerie skillfully folded and stored in her large dresser. The television set stood dark and ominous on top of her dresser, while her large mirror reflected the small pictures around the room. Cathy and I looked around the room, the two of us beamed with pride. We were eager to have Mom see her new abode.

Val, the director of The Bridge at the time, required Mom to be under a hospice program. Unbeknownst to me, she had been in contact with the Life Care Facility staff, requesting their doctor's Hospice company be contacted. "With hospice care in place," Val told me, "the amount of assistance your Mom will require from The Bridge staff will be less and consequently, we can keep the monthly cost lower for you." Evidently, the cost of living at The Bridge was based on the amount of care Mom required, along with the regular room rent.

"Hospice is one of the most underutilized programs we have for many of our residents," said Val. "Most people think hospice is a place where you go to die, and that myth has been perpetuated through society. It is true that hospice does have a facility, but it also is a program of palliative care for the terminally ill."

"Yes," I said, "I have always thought of hospice as a facility until my Mom needed help taking care of my step-father when he was dying of cancer. They came to the house to help her care for him when she was thoroughly exhausted," I explained. "It really helped her out, and they were there when my step father passed away. How will hospice help Mom now?" I asked.

"Well, they do provide respite care, but at The Bridge your Mom will have weekly visits from the hospice nurse as well as someone to help her with bathing two to three times a week. She can also have a massage therapist," said Val. "Hospice will oversee all of her medications and healthcare needs, which eliminates the need for our staff to do those things for her."

The next morning I met with Dr. Minaj from the Life Care Facility. He stated, "Your mother has lost a lot of weight here. I believe she is down to eighty-six pounds, and will definitely qualify for hospice services," he told me. "Since I have seen this tremendous decline in her health, it is a good idea to have her in a hospice program. I will contact them, and have them bring the paperwork for you to sign this afternoon."

Following directions, I waited for Annelise from Infinity Hospice that Friday afternoon. She brought the paperwork over to the Life Care Facility, and sat with me at a large round table explaining all of the paperwork I had to sign. This is what I thought was the final hoop to get Mom admitted to The Bridge. Annelise went over each piece of paper in the large packet of information. She gave me her phone number in case I had any questions over the weekend. She told me a wheelchair would be delivered, along with Depends, a bedside commode, a shower seat, and even a hospital bed, if necessary. I signed the paperwork and felt we had everything in place in order to transfer Mom to her new assisted living at The Bridge.

Mom chose a purple sweat suit to wear to make the transfer to her new home. She hadn't worn any of her own clothes for five weeks, so this was a big deal. As I assisted her with getting her arms into the sweatshirt, I was also trying to contact the front desk to let them know we needed a wheelchair brought to her room. I felt like I was juggling an active toddler while talking on the phone. Mom was so excited to get out of that nursing home; and she was even more anxious about where she was going.

Once the wheelchair arrived, a nurse helped me maneuver Mom into it, first swinging her feet over the side of the bed, then helping her to stand up. She was unsteady on her feet, and was relieved when she could turn her body toward the seat of the wheelchair and plopped down. As I rolled the wheelchair through the long hallways toward the foyer, Mom's eyes were huge, looking around at the facility she had never really seen. We were both giddy with excitement to be leaving.

When the ambulance came around the corner and pulled up in front of the building, we wanted to cheer. "I can't wait to get out of here," Mom said. We were surprised when they rolled her directly up into the ambulance, wheelchair and all. "Oh! This is certainly a new adventure," she said. "The last time I was in an ambulance, they had me strapped onto a gurney, and I literally froze my butt off!"

I chuckled, "You're right! The last time you had a forty-five minute ride from the Mountain Ridge Hospital to here. You went completely across Las Vegas."

"They had a really nice young man riding with me, and he made sure I was as comfortable as possible," Mom said. "How far do we have to go today?" she asked.

I laughed and pointed to the building next door. "We just have to drive from this parking lot to that parking lot," I told her. "I could have taken you there by wheelchair, but they wouldn't let me! I'll drive your car next door and see you in a minute."

Mom had spent a month in the skilled nursing facility; and she had been very unhappy there. To say she was anxious to leave would be an understatement. She was excited to see where she was going to go next, but apprehension showed on her face. Her sunken eyes appeared much larger than they were as she peered out from the ambulance trying to see her new home.

Cathy and I had chosen Mom's new home without any input from her, and I nervously explained, "We've chosen The Bridge for you. I hope you like it."

"It's got beautiful morning sunshine," Cathy said enthusiastically, "and you have a room in the front so you'll be able to see who's coming and going!"

"All of your things are in here waiting for you," I said as we entered The Bridge. Fear of the unknown was written all over Mom's face, her eyes huge and her lips pursed. It hadn't dawned on her that she wasn't going back to her apartment at The Echelon. She was just glad to be away from the Life Care Facility, but now she was going to a new residence; one she hadn't seen. I assured her we had taken great care in choosing The Bridge. "I just know you'll like it," I said. "The dining room is very cheery and with the light, bright colors that you love."

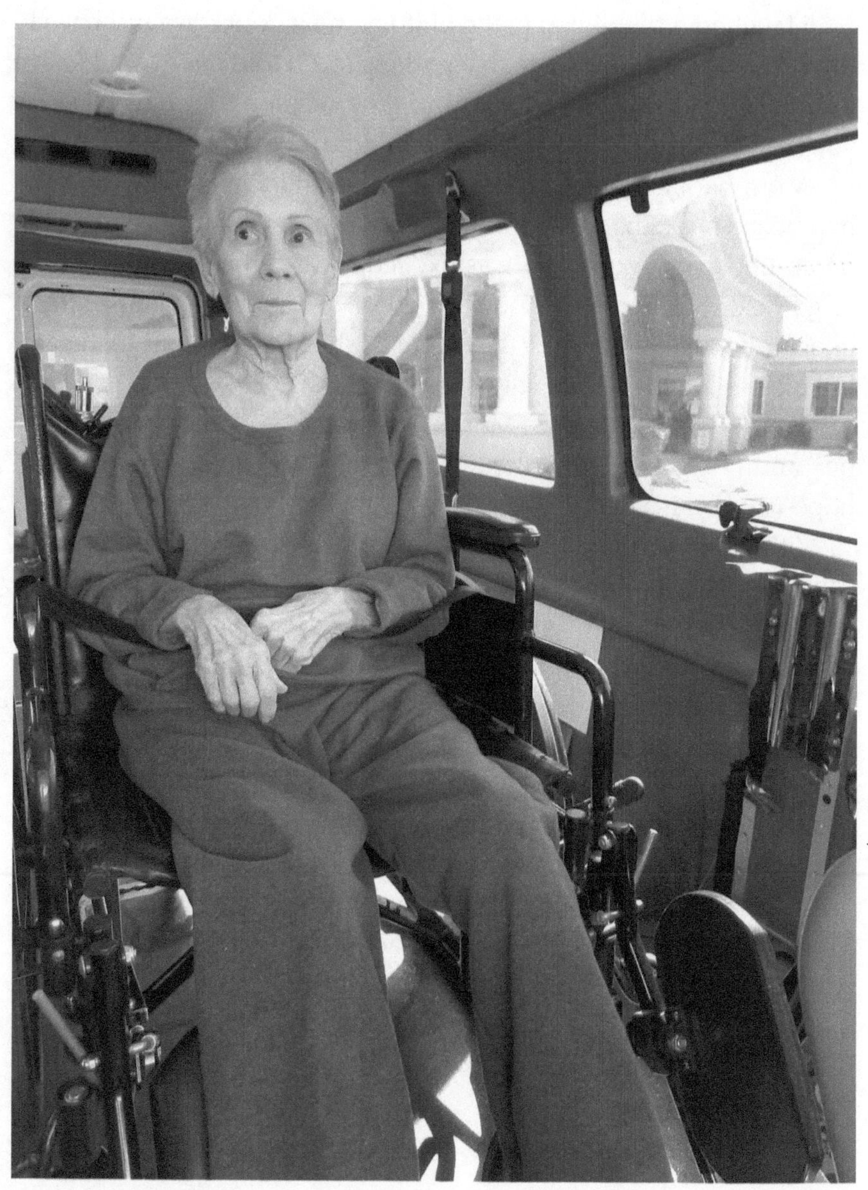

Mom in the ambulance on her way to The Bridge, April 1, 2018.

CHAPTER 16

THE HOSPICE GAME

THE BRIDGE HAD a Welcome Sign for Mom at the front desk. I pointed out the sign as I rolled her into the new facility. "Look Mom, it says, 'Welcome Connie Mears' on this cute little sign." There was also a lovely lavender wreath hung on the door to her room.

"Lavender is my favorite," said Mom. "My grandma always had lavender in her apron pockets, and when I went to her house, she always smelled like lavender."

I smiled. "This wreath will remind you of your grandma every time you enter." I pushed Mom's wheelchair over the threshold of her new room. "We're home," I said.

After pushing Mom's wheelchair over to her recliner, together we managed to get her out of the wheelchair and into the recliner. Getting her settled in her familiar comfy chair, I heaved a sigh of relief.

Mom looked around the room. "You did all this?" she asked. Cathy and I beamed.

"Yup," said Cathy, nodding yes.

"We wanted to make it look as much like your room at The Echelon as possible," I told her.

Tears welled up in Mom's eyes as she looked up at me from her recliner, "I'm not ever going to get to go back to The Echelon, am I?" she asked. A sad forlorn look moved across her face. It was as if a shadow had crept across the room.

"Probably not," I said, wanting to bend down and give her a hug.

"You mean I'll never get to see my friends at The Echelon again?" she asked.

"Oh, we can go over there for lunch sometime," I assured her, which brought a calmer look to her face.

Cathy piped in, "And we put everything that didn't fit in here into a storage unit for you, so if there's anything you want, we can go get it for you."

"This is nice," Mom said, her voice almost a whisper as tears again welled up in her eyes. She was a strong woman, and was determined to boldly face her future. She didn't let the tears fall, but a feeling of melancholy settled over the room.

Mom moved into The Bridge on Sunday, April 1, and on Monday, April 2nd, the Infinity Hospice nurse contacted me to say Mom was no longer qualified for their hospice program. "What?" I exclaimed, shocked by this news. "I just talked to the doctor two days ago, and he was the one who authorized her to be in this hospice program. I just signed all of your paperwork on Friday. Now on Monday you're telling me she isn't authorized to be in your program?" I was stunned. I was trying to keep my voice from yelling.

I explained the situation to Mom who was also shocked. "Don't I need to be on hospice to stay here?" she asked.

"I thought so," I told her, "I'm going to the office to talk to Val."

Explaining to Val the telephone conversation I'd just received, she said, "The Bridge requires your Mom to have hospice, you're right, but the doctor from Infinity doesn't work with our patients at The Bridge."

"I don't understand," I said. "How can Infinity put her on their hospice program on Friday and call us on Monday to say she doesn't qualify?"

"This is all part of the hospice game," said Val, the director of The Bridge. "Since that particular doctor doesn't work with our patients here at The Bridge, he was able to get your mother into our facility temporarily. Let me give you the name of another hospice company we work with," she explained. "I think you'll like their doctor."

"Holy Toledo," I said, shaking my head, "this is crazy!"

"Well, hospice focuses on the care, comfort, and the quality of life for someone who is approaching the end stage of life," Val explained. "They offer routine home care, general inpatient care, and continuous home care or respite care. Your Mom needs general inpatient care for the next six months. We'll work it out," she explained.

"I had no idea," I said. "but to switch companies within a day or two seems crazy to me."

"Well, you filled the paperwork out to get your Mom into The Bridge, but what they didn't tell you was that they had to put your application through their underwriters."

"So Mom didn't qualify with that company?" I asked.

"Well, they want you to use the hospice company affiliated with our facility." she explained.

"You know they not only offer physical care to the patient who is at the end of life, they also offer spiritual, mental, and emotional care to the patient and their families. They look at a patient who has approximately six months or less to live, and they try to make the patient comfortable, but they like to have different hospice places work with different care facilities; and it probably has to do with the personnel and the distances they travel," Val assured me.

"Wow, I had no idea," I said.

"Well, they don't treat your Mom's disease," Val said, "but instead they provide her with medical care to keep her comfortable. Having a hospice program is less expensive than having to take her to the hospital when something happens," said Val.

"So she won't have to go to the hospital again?" I asked.

"Hopefully not. Instead of sending your Mom to the hospital where she would incur enormous expenses, they will just have a nurse or doctor treat her symptoms here. Let me get you the information for our hospice program," she explained.

"Thank you," I said. I left Val's office with another telephone number to call.

I was frustrated to say the least, and explained to Mom that yet another nurse was coming by to interview her for the Hospice program irritated me. Mom's patience was close to a breaking point. She didn't like dealing with all of these strangers questioning her. "Each facility appears to have their own Hospice doctor," I explained to Mom.

Contacting the new company, Procare Hospice, I made arrangements with their nurse Janet, along with their hospice coordinator, Kristy, to come to The Bridge to evaluate Mom. One way or another, I had to make sure Mom was under a hospice program to ensure her stay at The Bridge would be comfortable, and to help keep her costs down.

Dealing with two different hospice companies at the same time was exasperating. While talking to Val about the new hospice company, unbeknownst to me the old company had come into Mom's room and taken the equipment that had been delivered on Friday afternoon. We were now stranded without a wheelchair. That afternoon, I had to make a quick trip to the nearest medical store, and purchase a transport wheelchair in order to get Mom to the dining hall for dinner.

When we completed the paperwork for Procare Hospice, they immediately sent out the same equipment which Infinity Hospice had just picked up. Out went the wheelchair, bathroom commode, and shower seat; and in came a wheelchair, bathroom commode and shower seat! I could see the Hospice care industry was truly a game, and the game created a miserable hardship for our family. It seemed ridiculous to be exchanging the same equipment, but I began to realize each Hospice company was vying for Mom's money. It was a business.

"Who's covering all of this stuff?" Mom asked.

"I don't know," I said, "but I'm going to find out. It wasn't until much later that I understood. Hospice companies are management companies. They manage your Medicare funds when a patient has a life expectancy of six months or less. Mom's Medicare payments were now going to the hospice company to cover her expenses. The hospice company then became her management company, so Mom was no longer under the Senior Dimensions management program, or direct Medicare, she was under the Procare Hospice program.

Mom qualified for hospice because a doctor had certified she had only two, ninety-day blocks of time left to live, which is equivalent to six months. This certification was required in order to be admitted into a hospice program. Mom had to accept palliative care instead of any kind of care to cure her illness. As Mom's designated health care director, I signed a statement choosing hospice care instead of Medicare-covered treatments. Her Medicare still paid for any other ailments, such as the time she needed to see a doctor about her hearing; but for the most part, Medicare paid for everything we needed under her hospice program. It meant Mom's Medicare payments were being turned over to her Hospice carrier.

We paid a co-payment of $5/monthly for each prescription prescribed by her hospice doctor. If a drug wasn't covered by hospice or Medicare, we needed to be sure it was in her Part D, which was provided by Silver Script, another insurance company.

Medicare and hospice worked together, using Mom's Medicare payments to provide a multitude of services. Through hospice Mom received a weekly visit from their nurse who would check Mom's heart rate, blood pressure, and muscle mass. These measurements were documented each week to determine whether Mom was losing or gaining weight, muscles, weight, and stamina.

One day while checking the edema in Mom's legs, Dawn suggested she have a massage therapist come to visit her.

"I don't want any stranger coming in and massaging me. I've never had a massage before," said Mom.

"Well, wouldn't you like to have a foot massage, or maybe have someone massage your sore legs?" asked Dawn.

"Oh, that does sound good," Mom said, as a smile crossed her face.

"I'd like that, too. Maybe I can slip into her schedule while I'm here," I said, joking with both of them. It was good to see Mom laugh.

"I'll contact the massage therapist, and we can set up an appointment for you," Dawn explained. "The edema in your legs is going to get worse if we don't get something done. I know you're not getting any exercise," she said, "so you'll have to keep your legs up as much as possible. "

"I know," said Mom, "they won't even let me walk like I used to. I could walk before I got here."

"Well, we'll get you a massage therapist, and you'll feel like a queen," Dawn said.

"You have someone cooking your meals, cleaning your room, and doing your laundry. Now you're going to have a weekly massage," I said. "You're a lucky lady," I told her.

"I've also got these lovely compression stockings for you that should help some of that edema," said Dawn. "I'll bet the queen wears them, too!"

A smile spread across Mom's face, and she nodded, "Sure," she said, "I'll try it." As it turned out, Mom loved her masseuse, and later told me, "She's a magician. You can actually see the fluid leave my legs as she works on them."

Mom became friends with her bathing assistant, who visited twice a week. Her initial shower was not a good experience. The shower assistant forgot to bring a towel over to the shower, and when she turned the water off, Mom sat shivering in the shower. Her Parkinson's tremors took over, and she started to shake so uncontrollably, she scared the assistant. Neither Mom, nor the assistant knew what to do. Grabbing the towel, and hurrying over to Mom, whose body was shaking uncontrollably, the assistant tried to get Mom out of the shower. When she nearly slipped and fell, both Mom and the assistant were traumatized. From that experience, Mom refused to have that assistant again or have another shower.

When I suggested Mom try the big soaker tub down the hall, she wanted nothing to do with it. "It's the same thing," she said. "I'll just be sitting there shivering. It's torture feeling your body shake like that." She didn't like the tremors and the feelings it sent through her body. Instead, Mom requested a sponge bath where she could remain partially clothed and warm. As with any hospice program, their job was to keep the Parkinson's patient comfortable.

A doctor was available for questions, but Mom only saw a doctor a few times. Hospice also offered a chaplain's services, but Mom assured the chaplain she had her own church and her own minister who came to visit her a few times.

A music therapist was also available, and since Mom loved music, I thought she would love having someone come and sing with her. Unfortunately, Mom wanted nothing to do with the music therapist, the physical therapist, or the occupational therapist. She also refused to see a speech therapist, not understanding that all these professionals were trained to make her life easier! Fortunately, she enjoyed the nurse, the masseuse and the bathing assistant, and she looked forward to their weekly visits. She considered them her new friends.

Hospice took care of Mom's wheelchair and bathroom aids such as a seat for the shower and a bedside commode, even though she didn't use the shower seat or the commode. Those items took up space in the shower where they were stored since the shower wasn't being used, but those items were available through Hospice. They also provided a type of Depends and handi wipes for toileting, but Mom didn't like the ones they offered, so I went to WalMart and purchased smaller ones for her petite frame. Creams and lotions were also provided for bedsores, dry skin, and massages. The hospice program provided additional support for the staff at The Bridge. They didn't have to bathe Mom, nor did they have to fret about her fragile medical state.

Much to our surprise, Mom was removed from her current hospice program. She was considered to be thriving. She was gaining weight, eating three meals a day, and not requiring any additional medications. The hospice company, without warning, came in and took Mom's wheelchair. To Mom, it felt as if her car had been repossessed. In tears, she called me and luckily I was able to get to Las Vegas fairly quickly. It took many phone calls and much frustration, but we discovered there were many other hospice companies willing to obtain new business. Another company came in, interviewed Mom, and determined that she appeared to only have six months left to live. It was traumatic adapting to a new nurse, a new masseuse, and a new bathing assistant, but there was nothing else we could do. Over the course of two years, Mom experienced three various hospice companies. They each provided excellent care, and we were thrilled to have them as partners in her care.

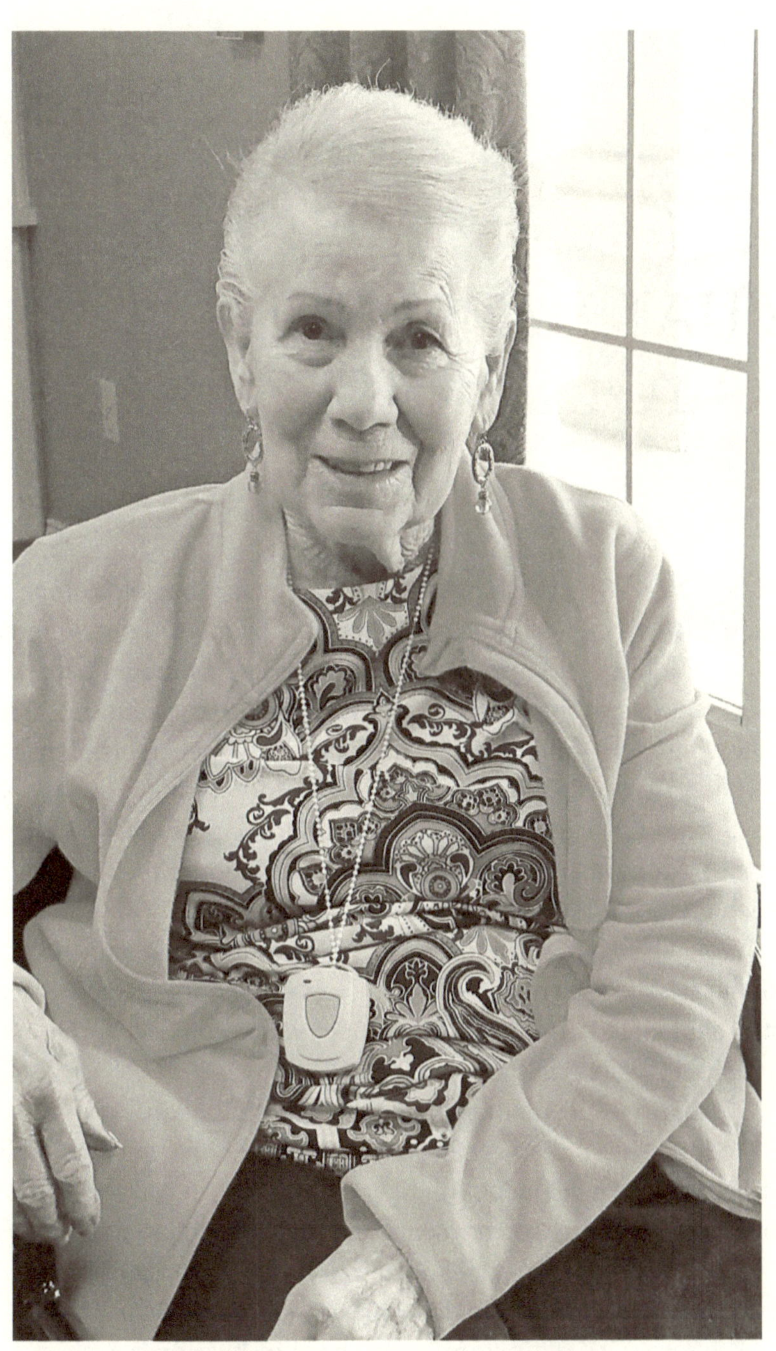

Mom in her peach colored sweater.

CHAPTER 17

WHAT HAPPENED TO YOUR VOICE?

I HEADED BACK to Washington, and Cathy went back to Minnesota. We decided to call Mom every other day, taking turns staying connected with her. "Parkinson's steals your voice," I thought after hanging up the telephone with Mom. Not only does Parkinson's make swallowing more difficult; it creates numerous speech problems.

The hospice staff approached me, "Your mother could really benefit from our various therapists," said the case manager over the phone. "We have physical therapists, occupational therapists and a speech therapist, too," she added.

"Well, she's already refused the physical therapist and the occupational therapist. Let me see what I can do about the speech therapist," I said, but I could already tell them what Mom would say, when I broached the subject.

"How can a speech therapist help me?" she asked.

"Your voice is already getting softer. A speech therapist would help you learn how to talk louder," I explained, knowing that a Parkinson's patient's voice not only becomes softer and more difficult to hear, but takes on a more monotone sound, eliminating any kind of expression or emotion in their voice. Sometimes their speech will sound hoarse or breathy.

"You know it's difficult for those hard of hearing people at your table to hear you." I explained, This would help you talk louder so they could hear you."

"I've never been a loud person," Mom retorted, anger welling up inside her. "I have always had a soft voice," she said, defending her inability to talk loud enough for others to hear her.

"Oh no you haven't," I argued. "I remember when we were kids playing a block away from our house, we'd hear you yelling out the back door, 'Caryn and Cathy come home for dinner', or 'Caryn and Cathy, it's dark outside. It's time to come home.' Your voice has always been loud," I told her.

Mom grinned, reminiscing about the times she had hollered out the back door to call us home all those years ago. "And not only that, your high soprano voice was pretty loud in church for all of your solos," I added.

"I don't need a therapist," she said. "I'm fine."

"I kinda' thought you would say that," I said. "Parkinson's attacks your vocal cords and their ability to vibrate normally." I told her. Even if she wouldn't admit it, I could tell she was facing dysarthria, a term I had learned when studying symptoms of Parkinson's. It refers to the softening of the voice due to Parkinson's; and it makes it difficult to carry on normal conversations, let alone have people hear you at a distance.

Parkinson Voice Project called Speak OUT! and Lee Silverman's Voice Treatment are two programs led by certified speech therapists who teach exercises and techniques to help Parkinson's patients improve their volume and verbal clarity. We weren't able to get Mom to try either one of these, or even allow the local speech therapist provided by hospice to help her. She was a stubborn old woman.

Mom's dysarthria was creating difficulty for her to communicate at meal time. It was frustrating for everyone involved, especially when she was trying to place an order for her meal. The waitresses learned to lean in close to Mom's face and listen carefully, often repeating her order back to her to ensure they understood what Mom wanted.

These changes in her speech brought on a deeper sense of isolation. One day, Mom told Cathy she was terribly unhappy at The

Bridge. "I don't have any friends here like I did at the Echelon," she explained. "I don't like who they have me sitting with at meals."

"It's only been three weeks," said Cathy. "You need to give it some time, or maybe you can try sitting at a different table," she suggested.

"They won't let me," Mom said. "They just roll my wheelchair up to that table, and I don't have a choice where I go. They just park me there," said Mom, her frustration growing. "I don't like being told who to eat every meal with. They don't read the newspaper and they don't know anything about current events," she told Cathy.

"Oh, I know that must be frustrating," said Cathy, trying to empathize with Mom.

"Plus," said Mom, "they can't hear me when I ask them questions about what's been on the news." Mom was frustrated.

"Well, when I get there, maybe we can change that for you," said Cathy.

"Oh, by the way, they are talking about how they have wine and brandy in their rooms. Some of them even have a happy hour before dinner. Can I get my wine and brandy in my room?" she asked Cathy.

"Sure," said Cathy, "we can ask Bruce if he can go buy you some chardonnay and brandy for you," Cathy told her. "Caryn can pay him back when she gets here."

"That sure would make things more tolerable," said Mom with a loud sigh coming across the phone line.

When Cathy called me to tell me about this latest development, I said, "She's already mentioned the wine and brandy to me, too. It's important to her. Good idea having Bruce go get it for her before we get there. That'll make her happy."

"Well if that would make her happy, that would be a step in the right direction," said Cathy, and we both chuckled.

Mom has always been capable of solving her own problems. When Esther, one of the residents passed away, Mom went down to her room and greeted her daughter. "I'm so sorry to learn of your mother's passing," Mom said. "Esther was always so kind to me. Do you mind if I sit at your mother's table?" she asked Esther's daughter,

"That's so sweet of you, Connie," said Esther's daughter. "I'm sure she'd love knowing that you were sitting at her table."

At the next meal, Mom told her CNA to take her to Esther's table, thus eliminating the frustration of communicating with other residents. Mom's joy came from watching the others as they entered the room for their meals. She quickly learned everyone's names, a little bit about each of them, and then gave them individual nicknames that she would share with me when I visited. I could write a book about Mom's dining room experiences and the residents of The Bridge!

Unlike many of the residents at The Bridge, Mom was not hard of hearing. She would often notice who could hear and who could not, noting who had hearing aids and who did not. Of course the hearing impaired residents spoke quite loudly, making it possible for Mom, who wasn't hard of hearing, to listen in on the various conversations. She was surrounded by many table conversations, and she quickly learned that many of them were talking about her. "How dare she sit at Esther's table so quickly," one resident commented. "Who does she think she is?" said another. Her audacity to take the table of her deceased friend unhinged many of the gossipers. The dining room was an interesting place, but as with any facility serving the elderly, it was also the highlight of her day. They all needed the socialization the dining room provided.

The Parkinson's patient's voice not only becomes softer and more difficult to hear, but it also takes on a monotone sound, void of any expression or emotion. As Mom began to deal with the new symptoms of Parkinson's one of the things I noticed was how her speech was becoming slower and more slurred. At first when I asked her about it, she said that it was due to her new dental work, but as the symptoms increased over time, I understood it was due to Parkinson's. The new dental work she referred to was, by then, years old. Although her mental faculties seemed to stay lucid, there were times when she struggled to find the right word. Cathy and I both attributed this to the aging process, but we also noticed she was beginning to ask the same question over and over throughout the day. Eventually we began to believe it was Parkinson's eating away at her brain.

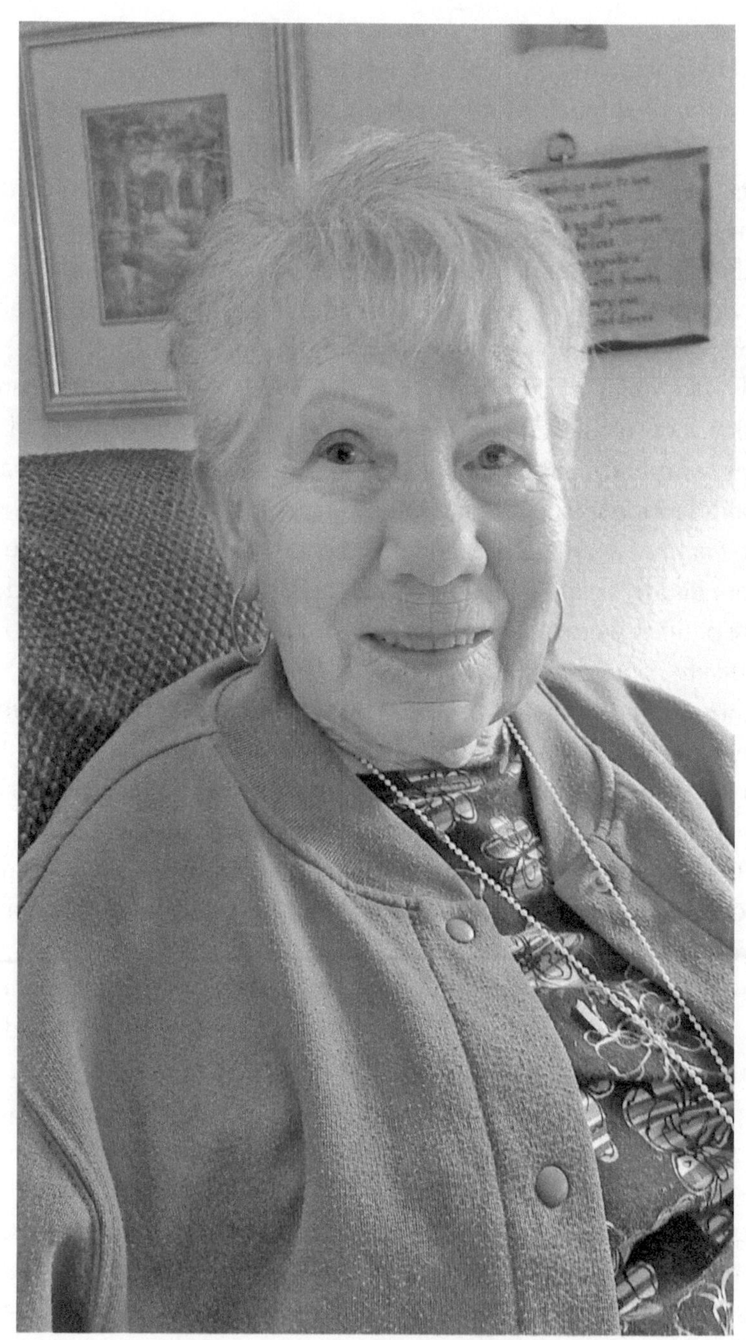

Mom after a beauty shop appointment.

CHAPTER 18

WHAT'S MY PROBLEM TODAY?

MOM LIKED TO contact each of us whenever she wanted to chat. She loved keeping up with her three daughters and what they were doing, but she also wanted us to know what she was up against at The Bridge. The telephone system there did not accommodate long distance calling. She could easily contact her local friends, but she was unable to make long distance calls. Her frustration was palpable, as she moaned about her inability to get in touch with us when she wanted to. Cathy and I took turns calling her every other day, but she was still frustrated that she could not reach out whenever she wanted to talk to us.

Speaking to Val, the director of The Bridge, I asked how we could improve Mom's telephone system. Val told me their provider was CenturyLink, and that I should call them to ask about their long distance program. Describing the situation to CenturyLink, they referred me back to The Bridge. They explained that The Bridge was a facility that had a Pit Code. The Pit Code was designed to keep other carriers from accessing The Bridge's phone lines, and suggested I get the Pit Code from The Bridge. So back to Val I went, asking for a Pit Code. She referred me to the maintenance man, Earl. He tried to work with me, but in the end, I became frustrated with the run around and decided to put Mom onto my Verizon account by adding a mifi system to her room. This created a good news, bad news situation. The good news was The Bridge had strong firewalls which prevented fires from quickly moving room to room; the bad news was their strong firewalls prevented the mifi system from working consistently. Mom's phone system worked intermittently, which caused her even more frustration. However, she was at least able to have a small amount of success getting me on the phone when she wanted. Cathy's connection wasn't as successful, and we soon discovered she was calling both of us every day, sometimes twice a day.

Mom's frustration was mounting. Unbeknownst to anyone, she had a bedsore and it was getting more and more irritating. Mom finally mentioned it to her nurse, and the nurse started treating the bedsore with a special salve. She also encouraged Mom to try sleeping on her side. That's when Mom refused to sleep in her bed. "The moment I go into that bed," she warned, "I will die. I can't stand the thought of being treated like a baby. Do you know they have people lay in their beds to change their diapers like babies?" she asked. "I'm not going to do that," she stated emphatically, putting her fist down on the arm of her recliner. Thus Mom began spending day and night in her recliner, which in turn increased the bedsore and its irritation.

Bone spurs on Mom's neck also caused her pain. There were calcifications on her neck. She had always told me they were from playing the violin. I had no way of verifying her logic, and of course, Mom was our medical aficionado, so we all believed her. It seemed the only time they bothered her was when one of the CNA's helped her get dressed or undressed. Mom complained, "One of the CNA's is being very rough with me when she comes in to help dress me in the morning."

"Oh no," I said, sitting straight up in my chair.

"She doesn't realize how painful my bone spurs are when she jerks my arms back and twists me around to help me get my shirts or sweaters on. I tell her she is hurting me, but she doesn't seem to care."

"We need to tell someone," I said.

"She's the same one who plunks me down on the toilet seat and it hurts when I hit my bed sore. Sometimes my bottom isn't squared away and it is difficult to pee and poop in that position," Mom said with a glum look on her face. "And once I'm there, I can't wiggle myself around," she said.

"Tell me who it is," I said, slapping the palms of my hands on the chair as I went to stand up, "and I'll go talk to Val about her."

"I don't want to be a tattle-tale," Mom said, staring off in the distance, seemingly calculating what would happen if she complained.

"You need to tell the office what happened. They need to know," I told her. "Which aid is it?" I asked.

"It's Roe," she said. "She's the one who is very rough, but it's what she said to me that hurts more."

I slowly sat back down in my chair, "What did she say?" I asked, looking Mom straight in the eye wondering what this woman had said.

"She told me that I should hear what the other aides were saying about me. She said none of them like taking care of me because I'm too demanding. She told me they call me the bitch in room 126," Mom said, and I could tell she was holding back tears as she pursed her lips and continued on explaining how her life was deteriorating. "I don't have any friends here like I did at The Echelon," she said, and then before I could say anything, she added, "Nancy has gone to a new place, and no one will tell me where she went. I'd go there if I could," Mom said forlornly, hanging her head. She was trying to be strong, but I had forced her to tell me what was going on; and her sadness was more than she could tolerate. She was no longer the positive Mom I had once known. I didn't blame her. Parkinson's had stolen the life she had been living, and now The Bridge seemed like a prison she had to endure. Her life wasn't at all what she had expected.

"Do you want me to talk to Val?" I asked.

"No," Mom said, "let me work it out myself."

Parkinson's was rocking Mom's world, turning things upside down. It had changed her ability to deal with life; and it had created a depression similar to what we'd seen when she lost her husband, Bill. The grief Parkinson's brought about, we hadn't seen for twenty-six years. Dealing with this disease was definitely throwing her headlong into a tremendous amount of grief. I was learning that the patient grieves the life he/she anticipated; and the family grieves the loss of its family member's once vital lifestyle. With Parkinson's, everyone grieves the past, the present, and the future all at the same time.

According to the Parkinson's foundation, apathy is also something Parkinson's patients face. Apathy is defined as a lack of feelings, emotions, or concerns. It can show up in a loss of cognitive curiosity, emotional lack of passion, and behavior. Mom faced apathy about the activities we tried to get her to participate in. She wanted nothing to do with group activities like Bingo or card games. She even found it difficult to attend the little concerts performed at The Bridge.

"I don't want to do any of those kindergarten games," she said, when I tried to get her to play Bingo. One day I wheeled her up to a table and encouraged her to play a card game with some of the other residents. That's when I realized how handicapped she had become. She struggled to hold a hand of cards. The muscles in her hands were starting to atrophy. Although Mom was as smart as a whip playing scrabble or word games, other residents didn't want to play those games. Their minds weren't as sharp as Mom's in that category. The easiest game for the majority of the residents was Bingo, so I got her to try Bingo a few times, but in her mind, Bingo was a kindergarten activity! I knew Mom wanted to socialize and make friends, but getting her to participate was difficult. She seemed very apathetic.

Besides refusing to participate in the various therapies offered by hospice, Mom was now refusing to participate in the social activities offered on a daily basis. We began to think her apathy might be a sign of depression. We had forgotten that she had lived alone for the past twenty-five years and had basically become somewhat of a hermit. She seemed to enjoy her alone time, or did she?

One day Mom said to one of the visiting nurses, "I don't know why God has even kept me here on this Earth. I'm no use to anyone," she said, staring the nurse in the eye, with a sadness wafting through her voice like a melancholy song.

The nurse replied in a very understanding voice, "Oh Connie! God isn't finished with you yet," she said. "I have a feeling he's put you right here, right now, for a very special purpose."

"What on earth could that be?' Mom asked sarcastically.

"I think you are here to help a lot of people learn patience," I interjected into their conversation. "You are in the midst of so many people who need to learn how to care for others; and you can help them understand what you are going through. You know you said you think these caregivers need to learn what it's like to be sitting in a wheelchair waiting for someone to come and help them," I added. "Maybe that's your purpose."

"Well, I sure wish the caregivers would have to sit in a wheelchair for a whole day and go through what I'm going through being lifted in and out of this chair," Mom said.

"There you go, Connie," said the nurse. "God's still got big plans for you. You are helping those around you learn about Parkinson's, and what it's like to be confined to a wheelchair. God isn't finished with you yet," she said, smiling sweetly at Mom and giving her a wink. As she walked to the door, she looked back and said, "No more talk about not wanting to be here."

"You're the teacher now," I said as we both watched the nurse leave the room. "Your purpose is to help these caregivers learn about Parkinson's, and what it's like to be in a wheelchair. I know it isn't easy, but if anyone can do it, I know you can!"

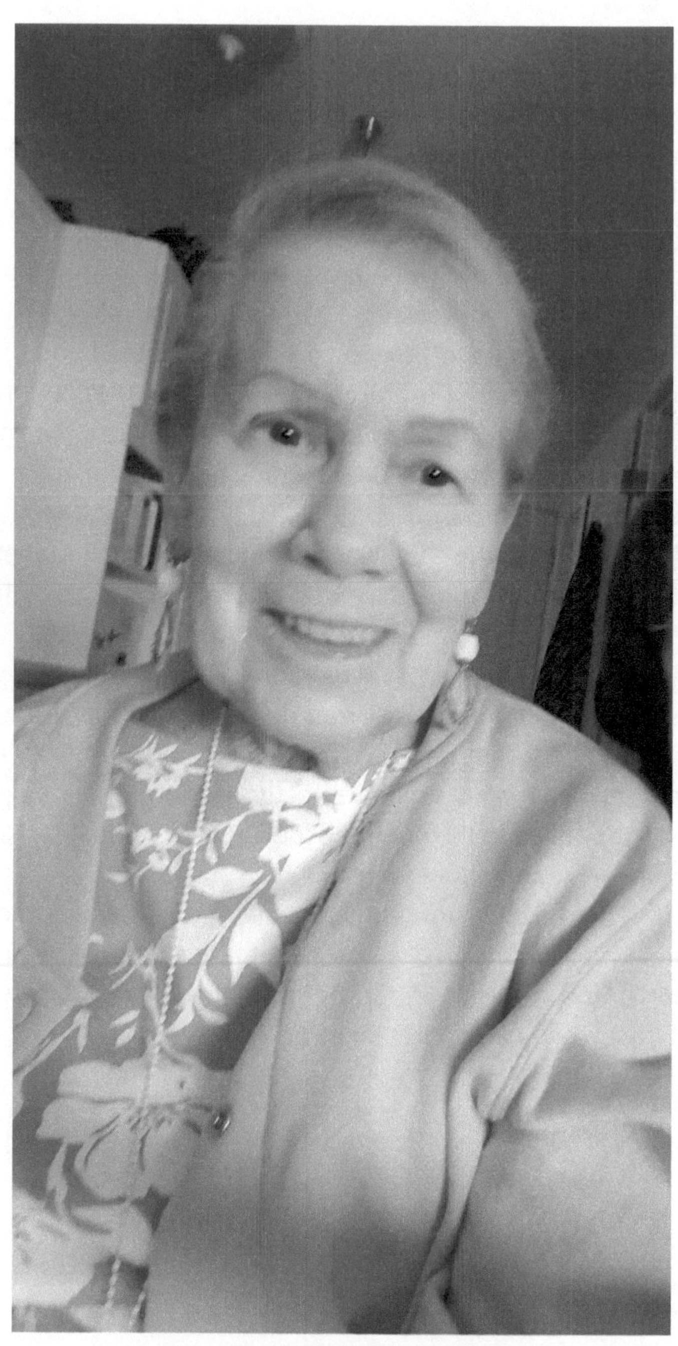

Mom in her favorite teal sweater.

CHAPTER 19

SLEEP PROBLEMS

MOM LATER TOLD me about her first night at The Bridge. She said she had been extremely sad and tired, and she had broken down, crying, alone in her room. Cathy and I had gone back to her old apartment, busying ourselves with packing up Mom's apartment, not realizing Mom was feeling deserted. She was so lonely.

Retelling what happened that first night, Mom's eyes welled up with tears. She began to cry. "I felt so alone," she said. "This wasn't how I had expected to live the end of my days. I missed my house, and I missed Bill."

"I'm sorry I wasn't there for you," I said.

"It wasn't your fault," Mom said. "I don't want to take advantage of your time with David," she explained, "But I just felt so sorry for myself. I was having a giant pity party," she sniffed, wiping her nose with a Kleenex.

"It must have been so hard for you," I said, my voice quivering with emotion.

"It was," she admitted, "but Nancy, one of the evening nurses came in and found me crying. She knew exactly what I needed. She laid down right next to me on my bed and she put her arms around me and hugged me."

"Oh, that was sweet of her," I said, tears welling up in my own eyes thinking about all the times Mom has had to face difficult situations alone over the years.

"Nancy whispered to me while she held me that night, 'I know you feel totally alone. Just relax now, and I'll stay right here with you while you drift off to sleep. You're in good hands here.' Nancy was the kindest person here," Mom said. "Nobody had hugged me like that for a long time, and she was right, I just needed that hug and I needed to relax." Mom admitted.

After living in her apartment at The Echelon for only a few months, then being in the hospital for a week, and then a month at the Life Skills Facility, Mom's world had been turned upside down. She was terribly frustrated at the turn of events. That night wasn't the last time Mom cried herself to sleep, but it was a night she will never forget. Her life would never be the same. "Parkinson's," she sniffled, "I hate Parkinson's. I just want to die."

Sleeping in a strange place had always been difficult for her, but now she wasn't even able to get up to go to the bathroom on her own. She felt trapped. She was literally confined to her bed, her recliner or her wheelchair. Waking up all night long, she had been agitated by the lights coming in the blinds and the new sounds she heard around her. "I couldn't even get up and walk around like I would at home." she said.

When Nurse Dawn showed up a day or two later, Mom told her, "I think the steroids they are giving me are keeping me wide awake at night."

Dawn said, "That could be a possibility."

"I need to have something to help me sleep," said Mom. "I keep waking up every hour on the hour, and I'm turning into a cranky old lady."

Dawn laughed, "Well, we can't have that now, can we? I'll let the doctor know you need a sedative to help you sleep during the evenings," she added, chuckling to herself about Mom's cranky old lady statement. As a hospice nurse, she had plenty of experience with cranky old ladies. As she listened to Mom's complaints, she knew she was dealing with a strong-willed woman. Even though Mom didn't want visitors seeing her in this condition, she enjoyed Dawn's weekly visits. Dawn became Mom's new friend.

Knocking on Mom's door, Dawn would call out, "Connie, it's me, Dawn, coming to check on you today." Dawn understood the fact that Mom couldn't answer the door. She understood how frustrating it was for Mom to get a knock on her door and no one would say anything. Mom was often startled by a stranger entering her room, but Dawn never startled her.

"Why don't people announce themselves like Dawn does?" Mom asked me one day while I was visiting.

"They just don't understand you can't see them, and you can't get up to answer the door." I told her.

Dawn's cheery smile was like a ray of sunshine when she walked into the room every Wednesday morning. Setting her medical bag on the floor, she pulled out her blood pressure cuff and put it around Mom's skinny arm. She listened for Mom's heartbeat as she took her blood pressure. In order to keep Mom from talking while she took her blood pressure, Dawn quickly inserted the thermometer into Mom's mouth. As Dawn wrote down all the data into Mom's chart, Mom quipped, "What's in your bag of tricks today?"

"Oh wouldn't you like to know!" Dawn said. "I need to measure every part of you," she said, pulling a tape measure out of her medical bag. She put the measuring tape around Mom's scrawny little arms, measuring the circumference of her upper arms that once were able to lift fifty pound bags of fertilizer for her yard. Then Dawn measured Mom's thighs, trying to help her determine whether Mom was thriving or declining. The two of them chatted away during their weekly assessments; Mom was learning about Dawn's family and sharing details of her own. Mom loved these interactions with Dawn, who was a captive audience.

Mom and I had a good chat after Dawn left one day. "The first night I was here, I had a Black man come into my room. He said he was going to undress me and help me get ready for bed. I was scared," she said.

"Oh! I bet you were," I said.

"I had never had another man undress me before, and this young guy said he was going to take me to the bathroom, and he would help me get into my pajamas. When he took me to the bathroom I was mortified."

"For someone who grew up in the 30's and 40's, I'm sure that was a shocker!" I said.

"But Cameron was so concerned about my dignity, and he spoke so softly. It was strange at first, but he was the best caregiver I've ever had next to Nancy!" she exclaimed. "When Nancy left to go to a different job, I was devastated."

"I wish we could have found out where she went," I said.

"I would have gone wherever she went," said Mom. "I hated the other night time caregiver," she told me.

"Yes," I said, "you told me about Roe. She's a big woman, if I remember right."

"Yes, she was always so huffy and rough. She acted as if it was a huge imposition for her to help me. It was as if I was interrupting her evening."

"You need to report her," I said, again reiterating our previous conversation. "How will the management know their CNAs are not treating their residents appropriately unless you let them know?" I asked.

"I know I should report her," said Mom, "but I don't want to be a snitch."

"This might be a case where you need to be a snitch," I said. "How many other people here are dealing with this woman's bad behavior?" I asked.

"Well, that's why I wanted to get a nighttime sleeping pill," she said, "I don't want to deal with that horrible woman in the middle of the night anymore." Mom was holding back tears and looked so forlorn.

"But you still have to deal with her in the morning." I said.

"Well, if they give me a sleeping pill at 9:30, hopefully I'll be able to sleep until about 5:30 in the morning. Then I'll only have to deal with her in the mornings, and not in the middle of the night. I hate being a tattle-tale," she said looking rather downtrodden.

I let the conversation drop. I could tell Mom was upset and near tears. She was fully cognizant of her predicament, which was a relief to me. She was able to verbalize her fears and any problems she was having. "At least you aren't facing hallucinations or night terrors," I told her. "Many Parkinson's patients are faced with those symptoms."

"Yes, I've seen the commercials for a medication to help Parkinson's patients avoid hallucinations. I'm sure glad I don't have to deal with that," she said.

I felt a shiver go through me as I realized our roles had been reversed. I was now the Momma bear protecting her cub. I remembered how Mom had solved her sleeping problem in the past, and I had to chuckle to myself. She knew if a glass of wine helps, then a shot of brandy and a glass of wine must be even better! Now Mom was wanting a sleeping pill on top of her wine and her brandy.

Insomnia is one of the most common sleep disorders faced by Parkinson's patients, while others face muscle cramps and tremors along with their insomnia. For Mom, the frustration was in getting to sleep and staying asleep. She also was dealing with the fact that she had to stay in one position all night long. She no longer had the strength to roll over, so turning was impossible. If she was cold, she would have to ask for help getting another blanket. If she was too hot, she'd have to ask for help removing a blanket. Luckily, she was used to sleeping on her back, but for everything else, she was at the mercy of the night time CNA.

Some Parkinson's patients have REM Behavior Disorder, an extreme form of sleepwalking or acting out their dreams. Some patients experience Restless Leg Syndrome where their legs twitch and jump, making it impossible to sleep. Some patients have sleep apnea, a form of loud snoring where the patient gasps and chokes for air while they try to sleep. Mom's sleep difficulty lay with insomnia, which was easily solved with a sleeping pill.

Since Parkinson's impacts the brain's production of dopamine and other feel good chemicals, it makes sense that many people deal with a lack of energy, and face mood fluctuations, sleep loss and depression. Cathy and I both thought Mom was showing signs of being depressed.

"You know, under the circumstances, you might want to ask the doctor for an antidepressant, along with that sleeping pill," Cathy suggested.

"Why would I want to do that?" Mom asked with a frown on her face. "I don't want to take any more drugs than I need to. Besides, the doctor told me drugs wouldn't help my condition," she said. That was the end of the conversation. Mom wanted nothing to do with taking an antidepressant, even though Cathy and I both felt she could benefit from it. She had figured out how to deal with her nighttime situation.

"We're just trying to make life easier for you," Cathy added. We knew Mom's attitude played a huge part in her ability to respond to what life threw her way.

"Oh, I'm just looking out for number one," she said. She was a strong woman.

"You sure are," said Cathy. "You're making sure you get enough sleep, stay as active as possible, and eat healthy," she added.

"And don't forget the most important part," she said.

"What's that?" Cathy asked.

"You have to have a sense of humor, because growing old isn't for sissies." she stated with a smile.

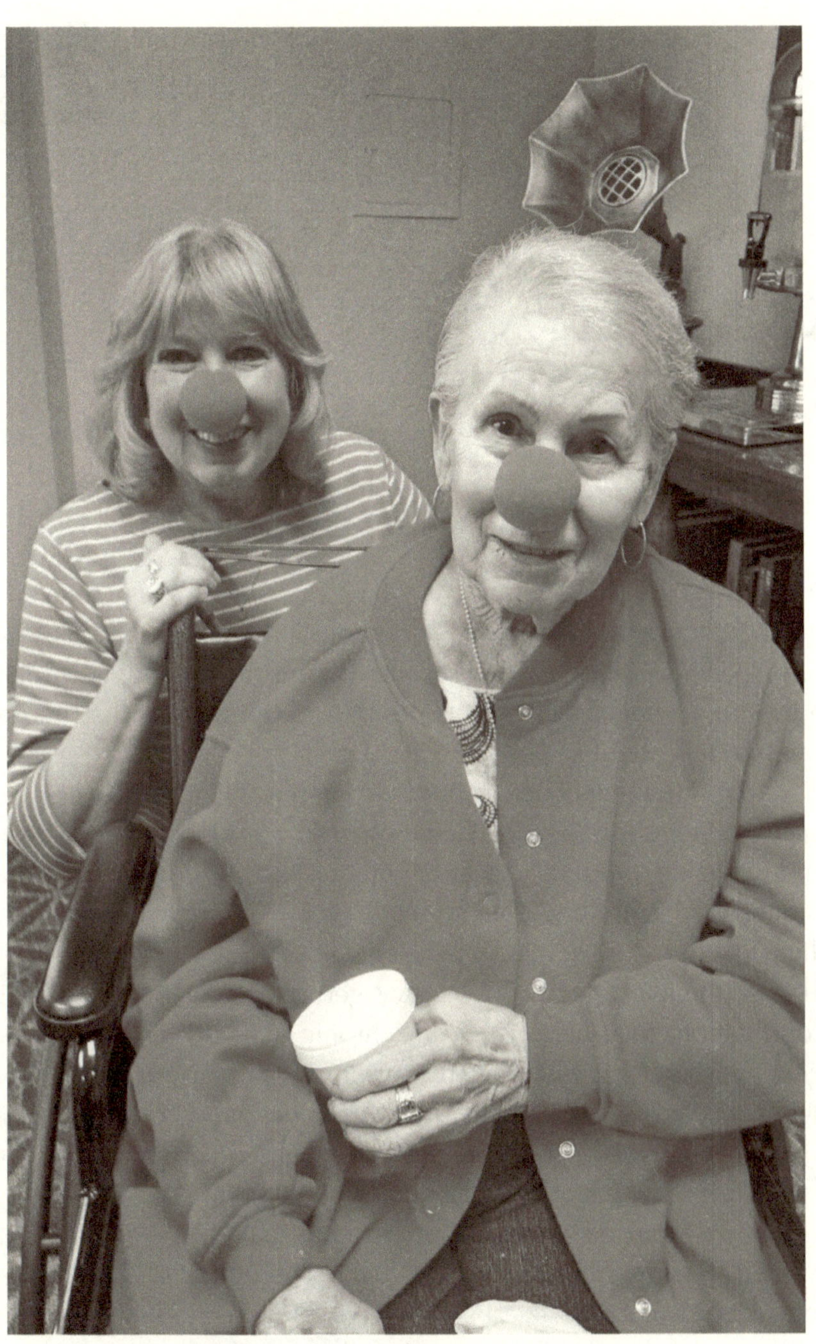

Mom and Cathy celebrating Red Nose Day!

CHAPTER 20

CONSTIPATION CONSEQUENCES

ALONG WITH THE sleeping pill, which eased Mom's nighttime trauma over facing the mean CNA, came constipation. One problem was solved only to introduce a new one. Parkinson's patients often face problems with sluggish bowels. It's part of the disease that no one wants to talk about.

Stools are the garbage of our body, and just like our kitchen garbage, our intestines need to be emptied. The stools are full of toxins and unhealthy products discarded by our body. When someone has Parkinson's his/her body has to work even harder to eliminate anything that is no longer needed. The bowels struggle to move the waste through the intestines as the muscles get weaker. Patients faced with constipation, may also deal with chronic gas and bloating. Other symptoms can accompany constipation. It can cause chronic headaches, hormonal imbalances, muscles aches, and rectal and anal fissures as well as high blood pressure, high cholesterol, and sugar imbalances. The gut affects many parts of the body.

When Mom discovered she was constipated, she immediately wanted to solve the problem from the inside out. She started drinking prune juice for breakfast and asked for a bran muffin. "Surely that will get things moving," she thought to herself. She chose to eat more foods high in fiber such as apples, pears, and salads, but nothing seemed to alleviate her problem.

Her next step was to tell Dawn, her hospice nurse, about the situation. Dawn in turn requested her doctor prescribe a stool softener. Much to Mom's dismay, the medical staff wasn't aware of Mom's susceptibility to drug dosages. Her body was small enough to require only a child's size dosage, rather than a full adult dosage. The stool softener prescribed was a dosage much too large for her child sized body, and the new stool softener subsequently caused her to have a huge bout of diarrhea.

For Cathy, who was visiting at the time, it was DeJaVu! Mom immediately called for an aide to assist her. Cathy, seeing the huge mess created in the recliner, sighed a huge sigh of relief when she realized the staff at The Bridge took over the care and clean-up for Mom. Two CNAs came into Mom's room, whisked her off to the bathroom, and then came to help clean up the mess in the recliner. They washed Mom and put her in clean clothes.

Again, Mom was terribly embarrassed. Although she was wearing Depends, and demanded to be taken to the toilet on a regular basis, this incident was mortifying for her. She understood the fine balance between constipation and diarrhea, and she preferred constipation. She no longer wanted to take the stool softeners if she was going to face this kind of diarrhea. She requested a folded bed sheet be placed on her chair to protect it from any future mishaps.

The staff wouldn't let Mom try walking to the bathroom with her walker. "You're a fall risk," they told her. "You need to have two people with you in order to use your walker- one person walking at your side and one person behind you in case you fall backwards."

Turning to me, the CNA explained, "It's just safer if she stays in a wheelchair," as she glanced toward Mom's wheelchair. "Besides, we never have two people available to ensure her safety," she added.

Hearing this, Mom's disappointment was written on her face. Her head drooped forward and she heaved a huge sigh. She was desperate for any kind of independence, and this statement confirmed she would have to continue her usual bathroom routine. One person would lift her out of her recliner, holding her up under her arms. They would pivot, then swing her around to her wheelchair and plop her down. After pushing the wheelchair around the corner to the bathroom, they would again lift her up to a standing position, and have Mom grab the towel rack for stability while they pulled down her pants. Next, they would pivot her again, lowering her down onto the toilet. Once the toileting was complete, the aide would help wipe Mom's backside, and lift her up off the toilet, again having her grasp the towel rack while they pulled up her pants. Pivoting again, they would plop her back into her wheelchair and roll her back to her recliner. Completing the process backwards, again lifting her up under her arms, and pivoting to swing her back into her recliner.

Sometimes it wasn't a gentle transition. It was an uncomfortable process for all parties involved. At eighty-six pounds it was much easier than when Mom gained twenty pounds from eating three meals a day. Her legs or arms often got banged up somewhere in the process, and once the CNA's keys hit Mom in the face, cutting her lip. It was an exhausting process for Mom and her caregivers. Unfortunately, this task had to be performed eight to nine times a day. The only one Mom felt comfortable with was her evening caregiver, Cameron. He was the young gentleman who became her favorite CNA. He was the only one who could comfortably lift her in and out of the recliner and on and off the toilet. No wonder she adored him. "Cameron always anticipates what I need," Mom said one day when she learned he was selected as the CNA of the month. "He's the kindest man I know."

We eventually encouraged Mom to drink more water, and purchased small bottles of water she could more easily handle. Someone would have to twist the cap off from the small bottle of water. She would take a tiny sip, thinking she was drinking a ton of water, but it was a step in the right direction. It was an ongoing battle to get her to drink more fluids.

Metamucil was a fiber product that we tried to introduce, but Mom was afraid of having another bout of diarrhea. With no exercise happening in her life, we encouraged Mom to eat as many high fiber fruits and vegetables as she could. However, we had to remember she was set in her ways. I soon found out Mom was a very picky eater. She did branch out from her usual peaches and cottage cheese for lunch, and began eating BLT sandwiches, and other things she could take apart and eat with her fingers. Eventually, she also learned to shy away from foods difficult for her to swallow.

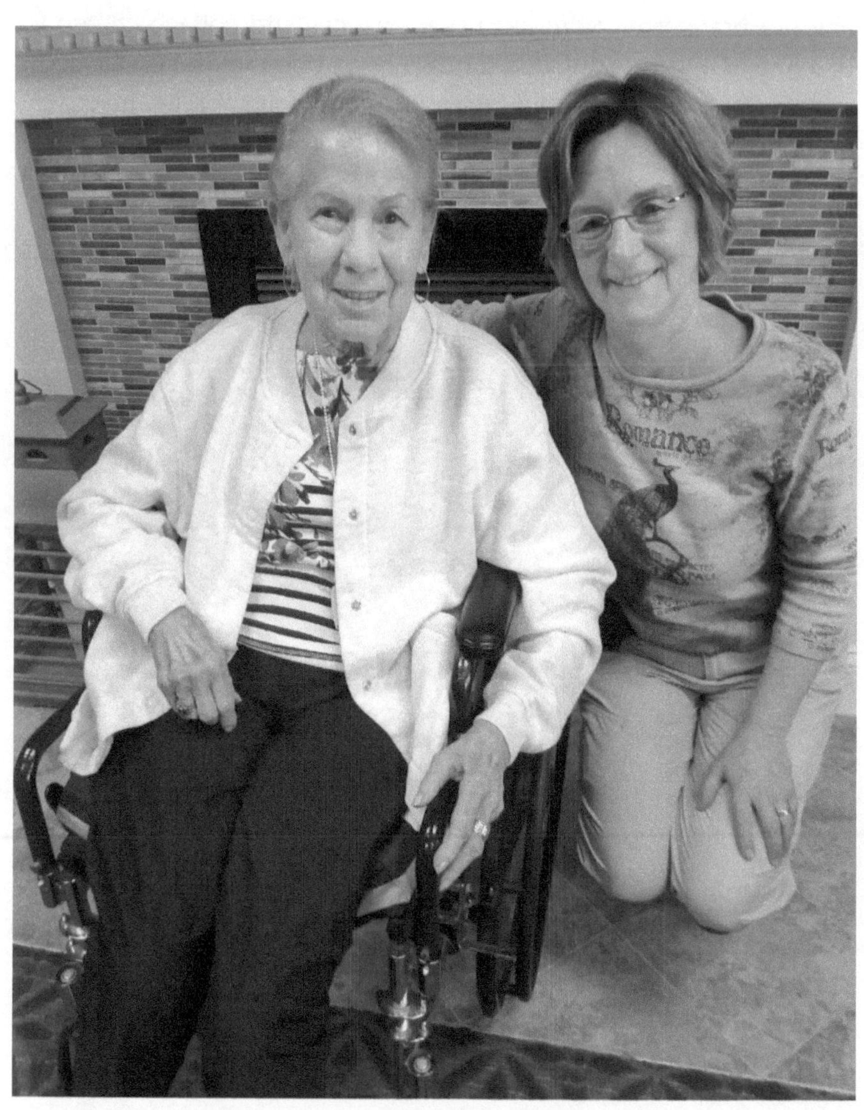

Mom with step-daughter, Anne Grimes

CHAPTER 21

EXERCISE IS PARAMOUNT

AT ONE POINT, I tried to get Mom to join me in simple patting and clapping exercises to help her maintain her strength. Sadly, when she couldn't do the simple cross body exercises, she became frustrated and shut down to any kind of exercise.

In order to keep their bodies strong, Parkinson's patients should engage in some kind of physical activity on a daily basis. A patient doesn't need to go to a gym to complete an exercise program.

When Anne, my step-sister, would visit, she would enjoy long walks with Mom. Their walks always involved long chats, while Anne, a nurse specializing in cardiac rehab, would share her expertise with Mom. When Mom was eighty, Anne noticed the decline in Mom's ability to walk, but during the early stages of Parkinson's, most patients can challenge their body to do more vigorous exercises.

"There are a number of exercises that help build up strength in the upper and lower extremities," said Jillian, my daughter who is a physical therapist. "Grandma can do push ups against a wall for arm strength and chair squats will help build up her quad muscles," she said. "Walking as much as possible will build up the cardiovascular system, but you have to remember to only walk as fast as you can while carrying on a conversation," Jill added.

"That's what I did when I was recovering from my heart surgery,"

I said. "I started a walking program where I walked three times a day. Each time I added a minute to my walks until I was walking fifteen minutes three times a day," I told her.

"Sadly, Grandma has progressed to the point where any movements have to be adapted," said Jillian. "For instance, she could form a bridge by lying on her bed, and lifting her buttocks off the mattress. Then she could hold that position for ten seconds before lowering her butt back down. If she can do that, she could try three sets of ten repetitions to increase her leg strength," Jill told me.

"Grandma is beyond jogging in place, but it would have been a good exercise for her in the early stages of Parkinson's," said Jillian, demonstrating with a chair next to her for safety and balance. "Just pretend you're running," she said. "It helps to have music playing. Some Parkinson's patients still enjoy dancing, too. Anything to keep their bodies moving will benefit their cardiovascular system," she added.

"But grandma can't stand or sit anymore," I told Jillian. "What can she do?"

"Chair exercises are really helpful," Jillian told me.

"I just discovered chair exercises," I told her. "We call it chair stretch," I said, as I demonstrated grabbing the back of the chair and twisting my trunk around in the opposite direction.

"Yes, you can also do the trunk twists laying on the floor," said Jillian. "Just stretch your arms out to your side and gently turn your head to the side and lower your legs in the opposite direction. You can hold that stretch for thirty seconds, and then switch sides, turning your head in the opposite direction and lowering your knees to the other side," she said.

"I wish I was here to help Grandma," Jillian said. "It often helps to have someone exercise with you. First because it is always fun to exercise with someone, and second because it creates a safer environment. I know I could talk Grandma into trying some of these if I were around more. I wish she would let a physical therapist come in and help her."

"I do, too," I said. "I even looked up a Parkinson's Foundation Youtube site which has tons of free exercise videos, but do you think I could get her to try any of these things?" I asked.

"I know," said Jillian. "She's rather stubborn! Those videos will help so many Parkinson's patients. You can mix up the routine, too, so you don't get bored doing the same exercises everyday," she said.

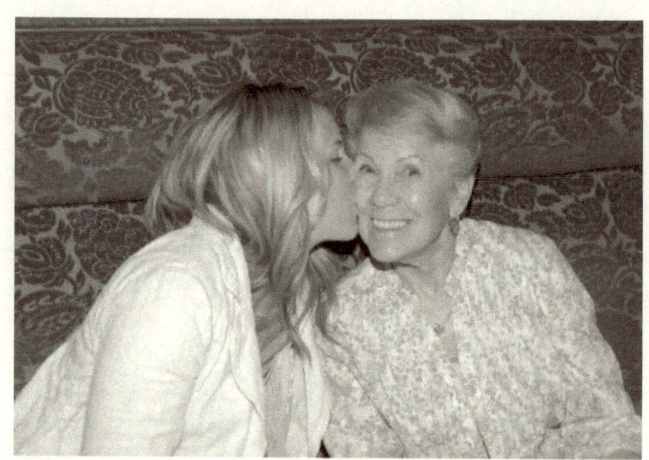

Mom with Granddaughter, Dr. Jillian Mears DPT.

CHAPTER 22

ANOTHER MASSAGE, ANOTHER VISITOR

AS THE MASSAGE therapist worked, Mom sighed. "This is heaven," she said, adding, "Caryn, I'd like you to meet my angel, Jackie." Mom introduced her masseuse who had just removed Mom's slippers and was gently removing her socks.

"Hello," I said, smiling at the masseuse who was rubbing cream on Mom's legs. "As you can see, Mom looks forward to having you visit every Tuesday morning," I said.

"You should see what she does," Mom chittered. "It's like magic," she said excitedly. "You can actually watch the fluid go straight up my leg, and back up to the lymph glands. It feels so wonderful," she said as she smiled at Jackie.

"Well, maybe I can massage your legs the next time I visit," I told Mom. "Then you'll love me even more," I laughed. "Everyone loves an extra massage," I said.

"Oh, I'd love that!" said Mom, grinning from ear to ear. "She leaves her lotions on the bathroom counter, so that will be awesome," she said, chuckling with glee.

The next time I visited, Mom reminded me of the lotions sitting on the bathroom counter for a massage. I went to get the cream out of the bathroom, and grabbed a towel to put under her legs. I sat down in front of her as Jackie had done. As I removed her socks, I discovered that no one was truly caring for Mom's feet. She had been getting regular pedicures when she lived alone at Seneca Drive, but ever since she had moved out of her home, she hadn't been able to go. That meant she hadn't had a pedicure for at least six months or longer, and her feet were in bad shape. Peeling away the layers of dry dead skin which were flaked around her toes and heels, I winced. Her feet had been neglected. I cleaned them as best as I could, and slathered a layer of Working Man's Hands all over them, making sure to pay attention to her heels.

Next, I lavishly spread a coat of lotion on one of Mom's legs. I began to rub the cream, sliding my hands from her ankle up to her knee in an upward motion as Mom had described. We both watched as the fluid left her lower legs and traveled up past her knees.

"That feels so wonderful," said Mom as I slowly kneaded her legs.

"You definitely need to have this done more often," I said. "The next time I come, I'll clean your feet and give you another massage." It was a perfect way for Mom and I to chat, instead of having me always across the table or sitting in a chair next to her. We were face to face and this position gave us a different perspective, closer somehow.

With the weekly visits from the nurse, the masseuse, and her hospice bather, Mom looked forward to her routine visitors. They had become her new friends, but unexpected visitors threw her for a loop. Being confined to her recliner or wheelchair, she felt trapped in her own room. Unable to move the wheelchair on her own, she had no way of escaping when friends would overstay their welcome. One day she asked, "Why do my visitors stay so long?"

"Well, when I visit someone, it seems odd to just come in and say hello and then leave," I told her. "So I suppose they feel like they have to stay at least an hour." I said, thinking about the times I had visited my friends who were in the hospital. "You can always tell them you need to rest. I'm sure they would understand."

"Well, this one lady from church came, and she stayed through the morning and then through lunch. She even sang to me and prayed for me," said Mom, her frustration showing through the scowl on her face. "I was exhausted and just wanted to close my eyes and take a nap." Her friend hadn't realized Parkinson's patients need sleep during the day. Mom was used to having a morning nap and an afternoon nap.

"That must have been weird," I said. "I'll send her a little note, telling her how tired you get, and ask her to advise other visitors who want to stop by to keep their visits short. She'll get the message!"

"Oh, that would help a lot," Mom said. "Did I tell you the music therapist called?" she asked.

"No, you didn't mention it. When is she coming?" I asked.

"Oh, I told her I didn't want her to come," Mom said nonchalantly.

I was astonished. Mom was an accomplished musician, so I thought she would enjoy the luxury of having someone sing with her. She wanted nothing to do with her. "I can't sing or play anything anymore," she said. "I don't like listening to someone else do what I can't do."

"Fair enough," I said, hearing my oldest daughter, Mollie's voice, in that phrase. "I thought you would enjoy singing with her, but I guess not."

"That's another thing," said Mom. "The hospice chaplain called, and I told her I had my own church." Mom was proud to be a member of the University Methodist Church, and didn't want to deal with more people intruding on her privacy, even though these services were provided by the hospice company.

"Oh, I'm glad they called," I said, looking down at my phone.

"Well, I don't really want anyone seeing me like this," Mom said.

"That's interesting," I said, "You don't look like you have any tremors or head shaking."

"No," she said, "but I'm not the same person I was when I was younger," she managed to get out between her pursed lips.

"Did I tell you I got your MRI results back?" I asked.

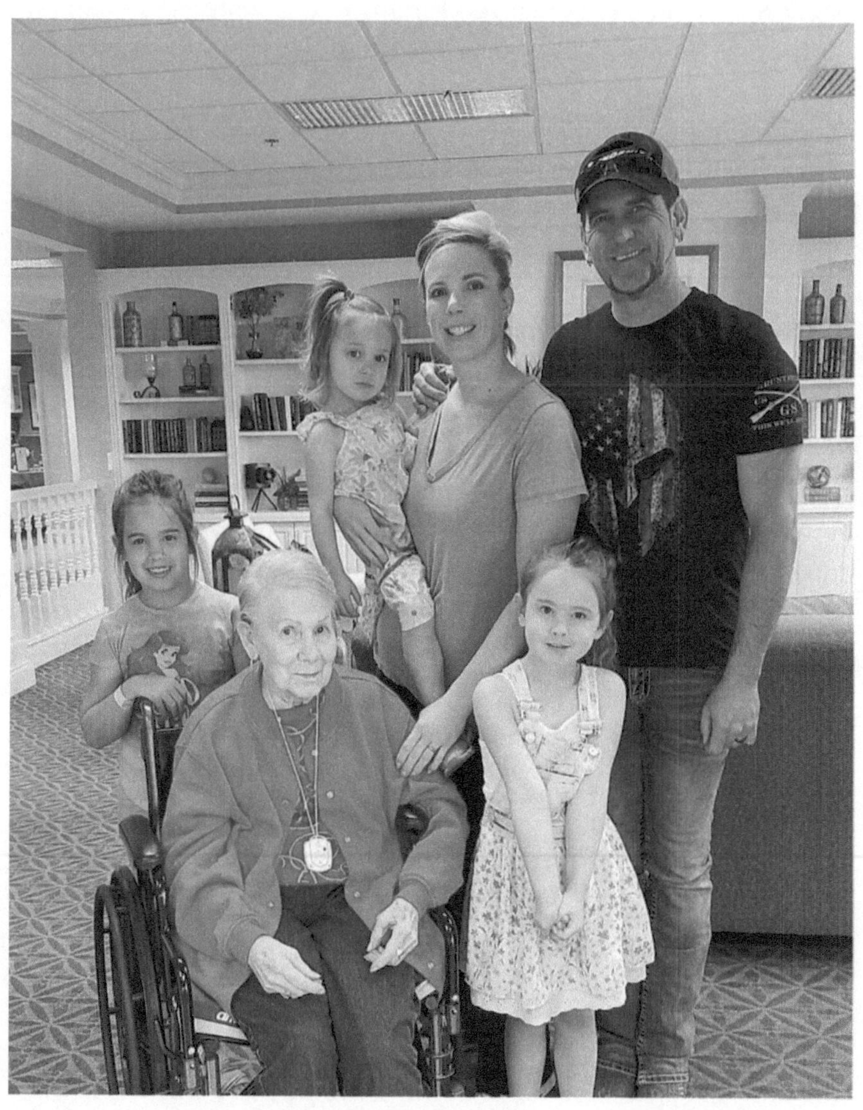

Mom with granddaughter Mimi, her husband, Rob, and great granddaughters Legend, Jupiter and Phoenix.

CHAPTER 23

THE TEST RESULTS

"YOU GOT MY test results back from the MRI?" Mom asked, repeating part of my question.

"Yes," I said. "It shows that you've had a lot of small strokes, as if they are eating their way through your brain," I told her. "It says you have supratentorial atrophy, meaning your white matter is shrinking due to the ischemic changes caused by these small strokes," I explained to her.

"Oh, my," Mom said. "I've never felt any strokes."

"It says that the changes in your brain are considered advanced for your age," I told her. "I think the time you fell off the toilet, you probably had a stroke. You didn't fall asleep there, but instead you had a stroke. I think you're very lucky," I said.

"Wow," said Mom. "I had no idea."

"Some of the smaller strokes could have caused some of your little falls. We'll never really know for sure." I said. "Each time the little strokes occurred, they were destroying parts of your brain."

"Parkinson's," she sighed, "I still can't believe I have Parkinson's."

"Well, this says that you have had many mini-strokes. It is as if Parkinson's is in your brain, and it is acting like a little PacMan character, munching away at your brain cells," I said, lifting up my right hand and demonstrating by putting my fingers together against my thumb, as if it were chomping away at something. "Parkinson's doesn't discriminate about which parts of your brain it munches on; sometimes it might eat away at the part of the brain that helps you walk; sometimes it might eat away at the part of the brain that helps you talk."

"That's scary," Mom said, trying to clear her throat.

"Yes, you're right, but what is even more scary is the fact that Parkinson's can eat away at the part of your brain that controls your breathing or your swallowing," I explained. Leaning in closer to her I said, "Just like that freezing experience you had when you were walking across the courtyard." I reminded her of the experience by adding, "Your brain forgot how to move your legs and you froze."

"Yes," she nodded, smoothing the blanket that lay on her lap.

"If your brain forgets how to breathe, that's not a good thing," I told her.

"That's an awful thought," she said.

"It sure is," I said, putting my hand on hers, "But these results are not meant to scare you. Remember the physical therapist at the Life Care Facility. He said no one dies from Parkinson's. He said that a death certificate never lists Parkinson's as the cause of death, but instead lists complications from Parkinson's as the cause of death. We need to do everything we can to avoid those complications, like choking or coughing, so we need to keep you strong and healthy," I told her.

"Parkinson's," she said, pounding her fist on the arm of her recliner. "I hate Parkinson's!"

"We need to look at the bright side," I said. "You are really fortunate that you don't have any memory loss. You're still one sharp cookie. You're doing really well for someone who is eighty-four years old." Mom nodded as I rambled on. "You don't have any hallucinations like the people in that commercial on TV. You're in pretty good shape."

"Parkinson's," Mom seemed to sigh. "I just can't believe it." She reached over to straighten the books on the end table next to her, and said, "I don't think I like those test results."

"No," I said, "hearing this is no fun."

"Can you help me call my friend, Joannie?" Mom asked.

"Of course," I said, reaching inside the drawer of Mom's night stand to pull out her little red address book.

"I need to tell her where I've been; and why I've been out of commission for so long. I'm sure she's wondering what's happened to me," Mom explained.

Joannie had been Mom's best friend since they were six-year olds at the Evangelical United Methodist Church in Wells, Minnesota in 1939. Joannie had been Mom's accompanist for all of her violin solos in high school. The two friends had been inseparable during those years. They had been best friends for over eighty years, and I knew it was important to explain to Joannie where Mom had been for the past six months. They had been calling each other every few weeks for years; and now Mom had disappeared without a forwarding address or phone number. Joannie was the one person who had known Cathy and I our entire lives, meeting us when we were born in Wells, Minnesota.

I gladly called Joannie and explained Mom's situation. "Mom wanted you to know that she has been diagnosed with Parkinson's, and her voice is getting more and more quiet," I explained. "She's been in the hospital and a rehab center; and has moved out of her retirement home into an assisted living facility," I explained. "We were just going over Mom's test results today, and she asked me to give you a call and explain what has happened to her.

"I'm so glad you called me," Joannie said. "I've been wondering what happened." We gave Joannie Mom's contact information at the Bridge, so she could continue to send Mom cards, and I passed the telephone to Mom. The two women had a lovely, but tearful conversation.

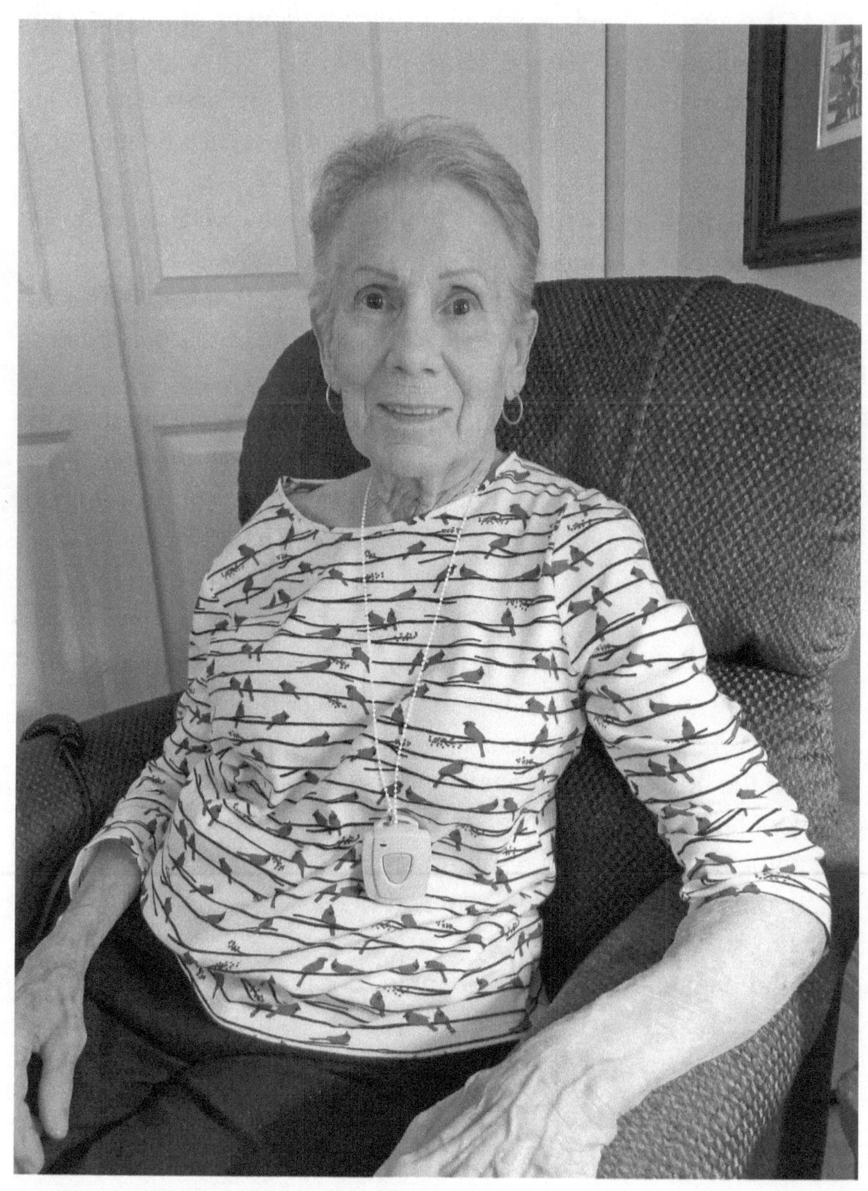

Mom loved cardinals.

CHAPTER 24

LOSING CONTROL

PHONE CALLS WERE Mom's only source of communication, and she tried to call often. One day she called to say she had a cold. It meant she was confined to her room, and was not allowed to go to the dining hall. She was alone, except for the CNA's who catered to her bathroom needs and meds. She desperately missed seeing the other residents. Meal time was the highlight of her day, where she got to at least see other people her own age.

"I'm going to come down to Las Vegas for Mother's Day," I told her. "It's next weekend."

Mom's jubilation came through the phone. She was ecstatic. "You've made my day," she said, "That's so wonderful. I can't wait for you to get here."

"Well, I could think of no better way to celebrate Mother's Day, than to be with my very own Mom," I said. "I bet you have lots of things for me to do!"

That was an understatement. Between the hospice nurse's visits; getting her car title transferred; disconnecting and reconnecting the cable TV; finding a long distance telephone carrier and getting her a new phone; straightening out her medications; mediating between caregivers and the staff over mistreatment allegations; and purchasing all of the things Mom requested, I found myself busy every minute of my stay.

Luckily, when I arrived, her cold was gone, and she was allowed to eat her meals in the dining room. Trying to help Mom make more friends, I went around the dining room greeting the different residents who remembered me. After dinner I even gave a little concert singing at the piano, and several residents came over to the piano to sing along.

Eating with Mom was an experience. She was such a picky eater. "I hate peas!" she said. "Why do they always give us peas and parsley? Why do they always sprinkle that green stuff on everything?" she asked, disgusted with the cooks.

"I'm sure they're healthy for you," I said, laughing at the thought of Mom getting peas to stay on her fork. I also knew Mom's aversion to peas, but I soon learned she had an aversion to many of the foods being served in the dining hall. "Why did you tell them you are allergic to strawberries?" I asked.

"Because I don't like them," she said. "It's just easier to tell them I'm allergic to them."

That made me think of the time she had the entire staff on alert watching for her to go into anaphylactic shock when the nurse mixed her meds into strawberry yogurt. She had told them she was allergic to strawberries, and the nurse had inadvertently forgotten that fact. They had checked on her every hour to make sure she was alright!

It had become a private joke. If you don't like something, just say you're allergic to it.

The staff did their best to cater to her desires, allergies and all. Part of our instructions to the dining room staff was to serve her food cut up into bite sized pieces. Eating with Mom often, I soon discovered this wasn't happening, so in order to cope, Mom avoided the difficulty of cutting her food up by ordering things she could easily eat with her fingers.

Mom always had a susceptibility for choking. Food, water and even her own saliva would often make their way down the "wrong tube" and trigger a coughing episode. Now, with Parkinson's, we were hyper-aware of the possibility of her choking. In fact, one of the therapists had informed us, "No one ever dies from Parkinson's, but instead dies of complications from Parkinson's," he said. One of those major complications is choking. Invariably, Mom would have a choking episode in the dining hall. The sputtering and coughing that ensued caused everyone to watch in alarm as Mom tried to catch her breath. A dining room assistant would come running, but if you have ever had a choking spell, you know you just have to wait for your throat to calm down. It was always a scary situation watching Mom go through these choking spells. Her eyes would turn red, and tears would stream down her cheeks. She miraculously avoided asphyxiation only to discover everyone was watching her. She hated this attention, and she hated being a spectacle.

One day, returning to her room after lunch, Mom announced, "I don't want this queen bed in my room anymore. It takes up too much floor space. Can you bring one of the twin beds over from the storage unit?"

"Well, of course." I said as I pushed her wheelchair over to her recliner. "I'll call Bruce. Maybe he can come over and take down the queen bed and pick up one of the twin beds from the storage unit." Mom wasn't actually sleeping in the bed anyway, so I wasn't sure we even needed it. It was there for show at this point in time.

"I've had so many visitors lately," she said. "Some of them sit on the bed, like it's a sofa, and I hate seeing them sit in these stiff dining room chairs. Can you also have him bring my green upholstered chairs when he brings the twin bed?" Mom asked.

"Your wish is my command," I said, laughing at the fact that Mom was still in control. "You know, I think I'd rather be sitting in one of those soft plush green chairs instead of these hardback dining room chairs, anyway," I said. "I guess Cathy and I were trying to save space with these smaller dining room chairs, but taking the queen bed out will give you plenty of room for those more comfy chairs," I told her. Mom was always good at interior design. "Maybe we should have consulted her first," I thought to myself.

"Well, I know you and Cathy will be more comfortable in those soft green chairs," she said, adding, "It will be so much easier to maneuver my wheelchair around in this space without the queen bed in here." Mom was right.

By the sounds of it, Mom had several friends stopping by to see her, so out of necessity, we wanted to honor her request. Changing out the furniture meant I had to call Bruce and my son-in-law, Rob, to take their trucks back over to the storage unit in the Las Vegas heat, get the twin bed and the two plush green chairs, and then bring them to The Bridge. Upon arriving at The Bridge, they would have to take down the queen bed and set up the twin bed, then take the dining room chairs out and bring the green chairs in. I was grateful we had put all of Mom's furniture in a storage unit. It enabled us to access everything she wanted. However, I was even more thankful to have two strong men to help with changing the furniture.

Mother's Day weekend we celebrated with four generations gathered together at The Bridge. The space created by removing the queen bed enabled the entire family to feel more comfortable. My daughter, Mimi, and her husband, Rob, brought their three little girls over to have dinner with Mom. She loved showing off her three little great granddaughters to the other residents. We were able to use the special dining room reserved for families, and Mom loved all the attention. My step-brother, Bruce, and I joined the celebration, which made it feel as if we were all back at 3398 Seneca Drive.

The greatest Mother's Day surprise was a phone call from Cathy, telling Mom she was coming for a visit the following weekend. Mom was beyond excited, grinning from ear to ear. She knew Cathy would help organize her dresser drawers and sort through the clothes in her closet. After all, Mom hadn't been around when Cathy and I had moved all of her belongings into The Bridge, and she didn't really know where half of her clothes had gone. During our visits, we did everything in our power to make Mom a happy camper; we ate meals with her, ran errands for her and often went out for special food from her favorite fast food restaurants.

"What would you like me to bring you?" I asked Mom one

afternoon. "Do you want Wendy's or Taco Bell?"

"I'd love a Frosty from Wendy's," Mom said. "I've really missed those."

"Your wish is my command," I said again, feeling like a magic genie in Mom's eyes. "Sometimes eating in the dining room isn't all that it's cracked up to be," I thought to myself, even though I was jealous of Mom having someone cook for her every day!

When Cathy arrived, she called me. "Mom's starting to forget stuff," she said. "She's asked me several times this afternoon where her violin is. I even pointed to it up over the cupboard by the door, but she still doesn't remember where it is."

"I know," I replied. "I guess since she really can't see it; she can't grasp the fact that it's there. She really is struggling to stay in control. She has a big job managing all the caregivers around her, but I think she's starting to realize it's a losing battle," I told Cathy.

"She seems to do well on the phone telling us what's happening on a day to day basis," said Cathy, "but I think she's becoming forgetful," she explained, relating several incidents that happened during her stay.

"You know she has been the queen of her castle for so long, it's difficult for her to give up any kind of control," I told Cathy. We both laughed about Mom being the queen of her castle.

"You've got that right," said Cathy, and the two of us chuckled together over the phone.

"Well, control or not, she is still very aware of what's happening to her," I said. "We'll have to see where this journey takes us."

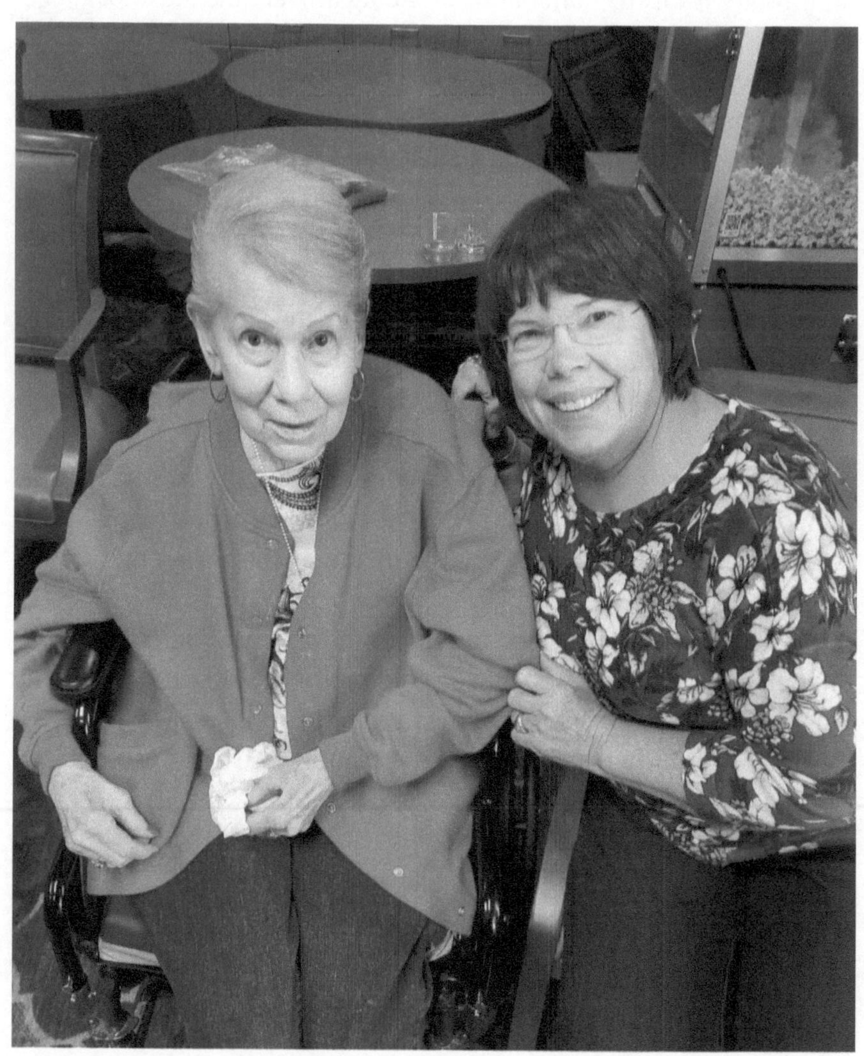

Mom in her red sweater with author Caryn Mears.

CHAPTER 25

WHAT DO YOU NEED?

TALKING TO HEIDI, a friend of mine who had been a caregiver in a nursing home, I said, "Mom is constantly calling the CNAs to take her to the bathroom."

"I know just how your Mom's caregivers feel. They're all arguing about who's turn it is to go get her; you get her this time; no, you get her, I did Room #126 last time." Heidi laughed.

"That's exactly right," I said. "I'm sure her poor caregivers are getting tired of Room #126." I laughed. I didn't blame them. They were getting tired of the lifting and transferring. Their complaints went directly to the nurses' station; and they promptly got the doctor to order medication for an overactive bladder. Mom was not a happy camper. She didn't think she needed more medication.

The next dilemma after taking the queen bed out of Mom's room was finding a twin bedspread that would look presentable. Having the bed out of the room freed up a tremendous amount of floor space. We felt everything was looking great, but we needed to find the bedspread. Cathy and I visited the storage unit, and after digging through several boxes, we couldn't find the twin bedspreads we had packed away. We decided it was easier to just go purchase a new one. The challenge was trying to find one that matched Mom's chartreuse green chairs.

Cathy ordered a twin bedspread from Walmart, but when it

arrived, it was the wrong size. Taking the bedspread back to Walmart, Cathy discovered they didn't have the size we needed. She enlisted my help and I scoured the Walmarts in my area. No twin bedspreads were available in the pattern she had picked out. It seemed like one of us was always on a mission searching for something to make Mom's life more comfortable. Eventually, Cathy found just the right bedspread; and life at The Bridge was coasting along smoothly, again.

Then Mom said, "I miss doing my crossword puzzles in the paper. Is it possible to get my newspaper delivered here?"

"Well, of course it is," I said. I was at home and had just recently canceled her paper, thinking she wasn't capable of handling it. "I'll call them today," I said.

Calling the Las Vegas Review immediately, they assured me Mom would have a paper the next morning. I didn't think about it anymore.

After a week or so, Mom called, "I sure wish I could have a newspaper to do my crossword puzzles," she said.

"I ordered it last week; and they said they would deliver it the next day," I told her. "You should have had it already."

"Well, I haven't gotten one yet," she said.

The newspaper office stated they had been delivering the newspaper to the correct address. That's when it dawned on me; they were delivering a stack of newspapers to The Bridge, but not to Mom's room.

When I contacted The Bridge, they confirmed my thoughts, "Oh," said the gal at the front desk. "I was wondering why we were getting an extra paper everyday." I had a chuckle over my mistake. I called Mom and explained my mistake. It had been three months since she was able to read her morning paper and do her crossword puzzle. When she called me the next morning, it was as if she had just received a very special gift.

"Thank you so much," she said, "I got my newspaper this morning."

"Oh fabulous," I told her. "I finally figured out it was my fault for not telling the staff at The Bridge that you were supposed to get a paper. They were wondering where their extra paper was supposed to go," I explained.

"I'm glad you figured it out! I love doing the crossword puzzles every morning," she said.

"It'll be fun to do the crossword puzzles with you the next time I visit." I told her.

There were times when we felt like we were playing whack-a-mole. One dilemma would pop up and we would solve it, just to be followed by another dilemma. Each dilemma seemed to require a shopping trip of some kind. One such incident happened when Mom decided she was going to sleep in her recliner. The recliner wrapped around her like a big teddy bear, but she was getting cold at night, so I ordered her a new blanket.

Unbeknownst to me, the air conditioning vent above her recliner had been blowing directly on her. When Mom figured this out, she called Earl, the maintenance man, and he placed a shield over the vent, redirecting the air away from her recliner. In the meantime, she received a brand new warm blanket, and was thrilled. She called me to tell me the details, "Thank you for the blanket. I'm assuming it's from you," said Mom.

"Yes," I said, "You told me you were cold sleeping in the recliner."

"Well, I had Earl come in. I showed him how the cold air was blowing on me, and he put a shield over the vent. Now the cold air goes somewhere else."

"That's great," I said, but was secretly thinking, "I wonder what the next dilemma is going to be." To mom I said, "You certainly know how to take care of yourself."

"I have to look out for number one," she replied, which we both knew was true.

The next dilemma came when Mom complained about her wheel-chair. She was uncomfortable sitting on the canvas seat. "It feels like I'm sitting on cold concrete," Mom said.

"You do sit in that chair a lot," I said, thinking about the bedsore that was taking a beating. I had tried out the wheelchair when it had arrived, and the canvas material felt hard. "You go to breakfast, lunch, and dinner in your wheelchair. That's about six hours a day spent sitting on that hard surface," I told her. "Let me see what I can do." I ordered her a purple gel pad from the medical store, which helped make her hours in the wheelchair more comfortable. It didn't alleviate the bedsore, but it did make Mom more comfortable. "We aim to please," I told her, as I zipped the new purple pad into its black pillow case.

It seemed every time Cathy or I turned around, we were trying to help Mom by shopping for something new. We both admitted to each other that we didn't mind the opportunity to run errands for Mom when we visited Las Vegas. It gave us a reprieve from sitting in Mom's room all afternoon; and it gave us a chance to do a little shopping of our own.

Parkinson's patients also face sialorrhea, which is the medical term for drooling. It can be a small amount on the pillow; or it can be excessive drooling that can be quite embarrassing. Initially, Mom's hospice doctor prescribed medication to alleviate Mom's symptoms. The patch seemed to work quite well, having it changed out every three days. However, as time went on, the patch couldn't keep up with the amount of drooling Mom was experiencing. Her new obsession was to tuck a tissue up the sleeve of her jacket and in a pocket. Before she left her room, she would make sure tissues were available. Cathy and I were often sent on a mission to purchase boxes of Kleenex, and at one point, Mom had twenty four boxes of Kleenex stashed in her cupboard!

We felt fortunate The Bridge had an aide do Mom's laundry every Monday evening. The only thing we had to do was provide the laundry detergent. Tide Pods seemed to be the easiest way to provide the detergent. The CNA who dressed her at night would throw two Tide Pods into the laundry basket. The aide who did the laundry would just pick up the basket, wash Mom's clothes, fold them, and return them. Another aide would put her clothes into the drawers or the closet.

Mom wasn't completely aware of what her cupboards contained. So when Cathy and I would visit, we always spent time showing Mom what she had in her dresser drawers, and closet, as well as the kitchen cupboards. I neglected to check out the bathroom cupboard; and one day Mom decided she was running out of toothpaste. I went out to purchase the specific size and brand. Mom wanted Sensodyne toothpaste in the travel size which was small enough for her to manage. Oh, my goodness, it was a marathon errand searching for that specific size and brand, only to return and discover she had several tubes in the back of her bathroom cupboard. This was a good lesson for me to check the availability of products in Mom's room before going on a wild goose chase! I did, however, learn that travel size products were good adaptations for Parkinson's patients. Their size was much easier for mom to handle.

The chardonnay and brandy were not dilemmas, but we wanted Mom to be happy. Each time we visited, we replenished her stash of alcohol. I also discovered a special brand of cookies she liked, and ordered those in bulk. Cathy, Bruce, and I were kept busy running errands for Mom, but we each enjoyed a chance to get out. Each phone call became a request for something. Whoever was visiting would get what Mom needed, and if Cathy and I weren't there, we were grateful to have Bruce available to help us out.

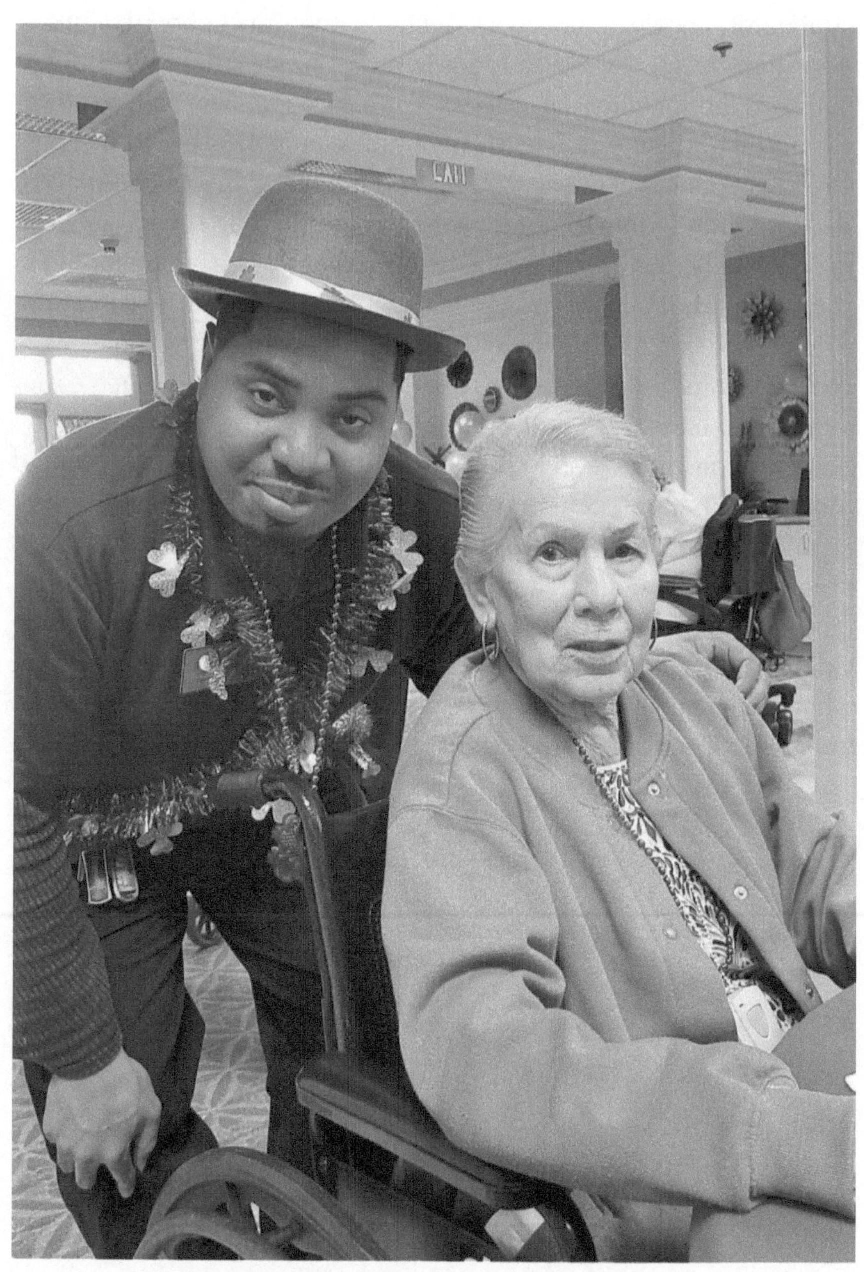

Mom's favorite CNA, Cameron Cleaves.

CHAPTER 26

MEDICAL AIDS

TRYING TO LEARN more about Parkinson's, Cathy and I read articles about the disease. One article suggested adaptive silverware, specifically designed for the Parkinson patient in mind. They were weighted and felt heavier and bulkier than regular silverware. They were designed to help people with a weak grasp, and were helpful to reduce hand movement. As I said earlier, Mom tried the silverware at one meal and didn't like the feel of the heavier utensils, but they may be perfect for another Parkinson's patient who is experiencing more tremors than Mom faced. We passed these utensils on to another Parkinson's resident at The Bridge. We always felt we were one step ahead only to be thrown one step behind.

Medicare provided a seat for the shower, but after Mom's first shower incident, she refused to use the shower, so the bench ended up being stored in the shower stall. Medicare also provided a wheelchair. The wheelchair was a godsend. Although Mom wasn't capable of moving it on her own, it did enable her to get around the facility with someone pushing her. There were days when she said, "I just want to get out of this place. I'm tired of these four walls." I would take her outside if the weather was warm enough. Otherwise, we would walk the halls. Each trip was fun reading the names of where each resident lived.

Eventually, Medicare also provided a hospital bed. You guessed it. Mom refused to use the bed. "As soon as they put me in that bed," she said,

"I know. You're going to die!" I said, finishing her sentence.

We didn't purchase a raised toilet seat, although Medicare may have provided one. We did purchase rails to go on either side of the toilet. They proved to be invaluable in allowing Mom to sit and stand when she was using the toilet. Unlike other residents, Mom insisted on using the toilet rather than going in her Depends. One of the CNAs told her, "I just don't understand why you can't just use your diapers like other residents." Mom was mortified. This CNA didn't understand Mom's background. I continued to purchase Depends for her from Walmart as the Hospice program did not provide the smaller size she needed. Mom was adamant about using the toilet right up to her final days even after one of the aides dropped her on the bathroom floor. She was lifted into her wheelchair to the toilet seven to eight times a day. The caregivers deserved an award for all the lifting they did for Mom.

The first medical aid we purchased was a cane. We took Mom to the local Walmart, and had her try out a few canes to see which one felt the best. We had no idea canes should be measured. While standing, with your hands at your sides, the cane should meet the crease of your wrist. Most Parkinson's patients use a cane for balance. In the long run, we did the right thing by taking Mom to the store, having her try out various canes, and allowing her to choose the one that felt right.

A walker was purchased for Mom to help her more easily get to her dining hall. When it arrived, we were all enamored with the bright shiny red color and the pocket which would hold her purse. However, we were even more impressed with the seat. We knew Mom could use that seat to rest if she got tired on her long jaunt to the dining hall. What we didn't realize was that the brake needed to be set in order to keep the walker from rolling backwards. Mom could have easily toppled off the sidewalk into a dangerous situation while using the walker without putting on the brake. There were a lot of things we needed to learn about medical equipment.

Walkers need to be sized to the patient's height. When sizing the walker, the patient should step inside the walker, and place his/her hands at his/her sides. The crease at the wrist should be even with the walker handles, and the patient's arms should be bent at a fifteen degree angle when he/she is ready to walk. The patient should then be able to walk in an upright position instead of bending over and pushing the walker. Not only is the walker selected based on the patient's height, but also weight. Mom's walker was much too heavy for her petite one hundred pound frame to maneuver, and after her fall, we discovered her beautiful new red walker was designed for a six foot tall man. Standing at barely five feet tall, Mom was struggling to maintain control over her gigantic walker. It was far too heavy for her to safely maneuver with the handles as high as her elbows. The four wheels also made it easy for her to tip over backwards, which she did.

The walker had arrived with no instructions, so we did the best we could. If I had known about sizing a walker, I could have exchanged it for a lighter, smaller model to fit Mom's petite frame. I also would have placed tennis balls on the rear wheels which would have helped alleviate the possibility of Mom falling backwards. At the time we received the walker, Mom had not been diagnosed with Parkinson's, so we were totally clueless.

When medical devices are prescribed by a doctor, the patient has a better chance of success with each device. We were only trying to make Mom's life more comfortable with our initial purchases of medical equipment. Once Mom had taken a tumble with the walker, a physical therapist explained to us that she was now suffering from PTSD (Post Traumatic Syndrome Disorder) due to that fall. She had tried to maneuver the walker, and failed. That trauma triggered her negative attitude toward other medical devices. If we had known about sizing the walker, we could have alleviated some of her trauma.

We later learned that Parkinson's patients have a tendency to not only fall backwards, but sideways, as well. Therefore, walkers can be treacherous during the later stages, but quite beneficial during the early stages of the disease. Once Mom was diagnosed, the doctor suggested a lightweight aluminum walker with tennis balls on all four wheels. "This," he said, "will help keep your Mom from falling backwards because she will have to lift the walker, instead of just rolling it along."

Now, just five years after Mom's walker incident, I discovered new innovations have been developed in the medical world. U-Step Walkers now provide maximum stability for Parkinson's patients. They are designed to have the patient step inside the walker base. This u-shaped base then provides maximum stability. The bars around the bottom of the walker are designed to help the patient stand erect while the rollers at the bottom of the base make it easy to smoothly transition over different floor types. The walker will not move on its own. The reverse braking system enables the patient to be in control of any movement made by the walker, unlike the walker Mom had received which easily rolled on its own.

Forward movement with the U-Step walker requires the patient to squeeze the hand break with the right or left hand. When the brake is released, the walker stops moving. This allows the patient to sit down on the walker without the walker rolling away, which is another detriment of the other types of walkers. The U-Step walker has been designed with a locking pin which can be placed into the back wheels to alleviate a backwards fall.

The most innovative development made by U-Step Walkers is the laser module and sound system. It assists Parkinson's patients who tend to freeze. The laser flashes a steady light meant to keep the brain continuing in a forward motion, eliminating the freezing episodes. There is also a sound pattern to assist Parkinson's patients to continue with their forward motion. With the laser and the sound operating together, the patients will be able to maintain a forward motion, eliminating the freezing gait. If only we had known about this technology when Mom was in rehab. She wouldn't have had to rely on her own verbal commands, saying, "Left, right, left, right," to keep moving forward and eliminate the freezing she experienced. The nicest thing about the U-Step Walker is the fact that the laser and lights are built in and the patient doesn't have to remember to do any self talk.

The U-Step Walkers are sturdy, yet collapsible. The seven wheels make it structurally sound, and the twenty-nine inch turning radius makes it easy to maneuver, even when in smaller spaces like Mom's little retirement home. Although we weren't able to purchase this walker, I would highly recommend it for Parkinson's patients who want to maintain their mobility.

Little did we know, our next endeavor with medical equipment would prove to be even more disastrous. Wanting to make Mom's life easier and more comfortable, I took her to the medical store to purchase a scooter, thinking it was the perfect piece of medical equipment to help her get to dinner in the dining hall, almost a half mile away. In the medical store, the sales associate and I coerced Mom out of the nice recliner she had settled into, and got her to sit on the scooter. She was very trepidatious, but as she shuffled her way over to the scooter and sat upon its black leather seat, she proudly smiled. "This is a start," I thought to myself.

"You can take it outside and see how it works," said the sales associate. "We have a parking lot right outside the door."

"Oh, no," said Mom, "It'll be alright."

"Do you like it?" I asked. "Do you think you could use it to get back and forth to dinner?"

Mom smiled.

"Should we get it?" I asked, wondering if this was the right decision as I set my purse on the counter.

Mom smiled and nodded, yes. Without taking the scooter for a test drive, we purchased it. It felt like we had almost purchased it sight unseen. I had trepidations and should have listened to my gut feelings.

The sales associate walked us out to Mom's car. There, he showed me how to break the scooter down into pieces that would fit into the back of our little Rav4. First the back came off; and then the motor was disconnected. After practicing how to assemble and disassemble the little scooter, I loaded it into Mom's car. Buckling Mom into the passenger seat, the salesman looked her directly in the eye and gave her strict instructions. "Be sure you take the scooter out into your parking lot, and practice, practice, practice," he said. "It's as if you are a new teenager learning to drive a car all over again," he told her.

Mom coyly grinned and nodded, as if to say, "I've been driving for sixty years; I'll be fine."

Arriving back at Mom's retirement home, I got Mom's cane and helped her get out of the car. As she watched, I put the scooter together and set it on the pavement. "Should we take it out to the parking lot to practice a little before we take it to dinner?"

Mom's reply was typical, "No, I'll be fine."

Not thinking, I accepted her answer. That was my first mistake. My second mistake was forgetting her fine motor skills had deteriorated. Fortunately, I recognized the two little icons near the key. One was a picture of a tortoise; and one was a picture of a rabbit. I laughed to myself as I turned the switch to the picture of the turtle. "That should solve any problems of Mom going too fast," I said to myself, hoping the machine would move at a snail's pace. Unfortunately, turtle speed would prove to be too much for Mom to handle.

Mom's eyesight was deteriorating, along with her depth perception, and I hadn't anticipated that a short jaunt to the dining hall could require so many skills. Not only did she have to operate the scooter in a forward motion; she had to stop the vehicle; and then there was the matter of staying on the sidewalk, which proved to be no easy task.

Now, you must realize this is my Mom. She told me she didn't need to practice; and she told me she could do it herself. I felt as if I were in a time warp, dealing with a stubborn two year old. "Okay," I thought, "she's been driving for a very long time, so she should know what she's doing." What else could I say? She was not a stubborn two year old, but instead was a stubborn old lady!

Sitting on the black leather seat, her feet resting on the floorboard in front of her, Mom turned the key, and the scooter lurched forward.

We were heading down the sidewalk towards the dining hall. Mom was driving the little red scooter, cane by her side, with me trotting nervously by her side ready to ward off any mishaps. It reminded me of my dad running alongside my first bicycle ride, trying to anticipate any mishap along the way. I'm no spring chicken, so I'm not exactly sure what I was going to do, if something did happen. Nevertheless, I can tell you, I wasn't ready for what happened next.

Mom started to tell me a story about a lady named Mary who lived at The Echelon. "About a month ago, Mary was driving her scooter along this sidewalk, and she went over the edge."

"Oh, my!" I said. "What happened to her?"

"She died," Mom said bluntly.

"What?" I said, "She died?" I gasped. The thought of an elderly woman sprawled on the rocks off the edge of the sidewalk materialized right before my eyes. "What happened?" I asked.

"Well, her scooter slipped off the edge of the sidewalk, and she hit her head on the rocks. They took her to the hospital and discovered she had broken some ribs which punctured her lungs. She ended up getting pneumonia and died," Mom explained.

"Well, you need to be extra careful," I said, watching Mom steer the scooter along the same sidewalk Mary had unsuccessfully navigated. I was petrified. Mom could easily miss a curve or overshoot a corner, and suffer the same fate as she meandered her way through the large courtyard. She was going extremely slow, but a thread of fear ran across her face as she concentrated on the path ahead.

Once we were close to the dining hall door, I jogged around to the front of Mom and the scooter, and opened the door into the main office. Mom zipped past me. I wasn't ready for what happened next. My maneuver left me behind her as she crossed the threshold, heading full tortoise speed past the mailboxes toward the main desk. Bam! Mom crashed into the main desk, startling the director who was standing behind the counter.

"Back that thing up!" yelled the director. "You can't drive it in here like that!" She glared at Mom, her beady eyes showing no mercy.

Mom was mortified. Embarrassed beyond belief, she put the scooter in reverse, wanting to desperately crawl into a hole. Unfortunately, the scooter's tortoise speed sent her zipping across the small foyer. "Bam! She promptly crashed into the wall behind her! "Park that thing over there, and go get some lessons on how to drive it," yelled the director. Her voice was curt and full of anger.

Mom sheepishly reached for her cane, as she gingerly slid off the scooter's seat. Her head hung low as she slowly shuffled from the reception area to her table. She had never been yelled at like that, and she was desperately fighting off tears!

"How dare she yell at me!" Mom said, as she plunked herself down in the dining hall chair. She was crushed. "I'm not a two year old that needs to be reprimanded like that," she said.

I giggled, and Mom looked at me. Through pursed lips she said, "It's not funny!"

"I'm sorry," I said, trying to hide my snickers. I felt as if I had just lived through some kind of a cartoon. Stifling my giggles, I played the episode back in my mind. It really was funny, but I felt sorry for Mom. She was devastated. Needless to say, dinner was eaten in silence, except for Mom grumbling about being treated like a two year old. The director did come over and apologize. She politely suggested Mom go out into the parking lot and practice. The silence that followed was filled with thoughts about our choice to purchase the scooter.

Mom, still sulking about how she had been treated, hobbled out to the scooter. I was surprised she got back on the scooter, but we both knew it had to be done. As we made our way back to her apartment, I walked behind her, keeping an eye on how she maneuvered her way along the path. Luckily, the scooter had a good headlight, since it had grown dark while we were inside the dining hall.

Again, jogging ahead, I unlocked the door to Mom's apartment, and held the door wide open. Mom drove the scooter over the threshold and stopped in the hallway, "You park that damn beast," she said, "I've got to go to the bathroom!" She grabbed her cane, shimmied off the seat, and shuffled her way down the hall.

Parking "the beast", as Mom now referred to the scooter, was more difficult than I had assumed, and I soon learned just how difficult it was to deal with the touchy mechanisms. Even the "Turtle Speed" was too fast, especially since I had no idea what I was doing. I felt like I needed some practice learning how to maneuver this machine.

Mom came tottering back from the bathroom, "You'll have to take that thing back," she said. "I don't want it. It's too hard to drive, and I don't want to end up in the hospital like Mary."

"You don't want to take it out in the parking lot and practice?" I asked.

"Absolutely not! Get rid of it!" she said, shuffling over to her couch. She plopped down, and sighed. She was emotionally and physically drained from her traumatic ordeal with "the beast"!

The sales associate graciously accepted my return, and refunded our money. "My Mom told me she doesn't want this beast," I laughed.

"She wouldn't take it out, and learn how to drive it, would she?" he asked.

"No, it was pretty intimidating," I told him.

"I'm sorry it didn't work out for you," he said.

"Anyone who can drive one of these things has my respect and admiration," I said, and I thanked him for being so understanding.

Thinking about our trips in the car, I so often wished I had purchased a 360 degree swivel seat. This device would have enabled me to swing Mom's legs around to the front or turn her to the side to enable an easier exit. This medical aid is easily obtained on Amazon. com.

By the time we discovered Mom had Parkinson's, she was beyond using a smartphone. One of the biggest challenges we had was getting a telephone that Mom could operate. She loved her little Cricket designed with larger numbers, and older people in mind. A smartphone can be very beneficial to a Parkinson's patient. A good App to download is www.mytherapyapp.com. It allows patients to set timers to remind themselves to take their medications, or to exercise, or even go for meals. It's a great help as a reminder for therapist appointments, as well. An Echo dot can also be beneficial, as long as the patient is near the device and their voice is loud enough to enable the unit.

Another App which helps Parkinson's patients is called, "One Step Gait Analysis". It is an app to download onto your smartphone which allows users to choose which area of their body they would like to analyze. It offers a free trial in which you are able to connect with a physical therapist, who is available at www.onestep.com.

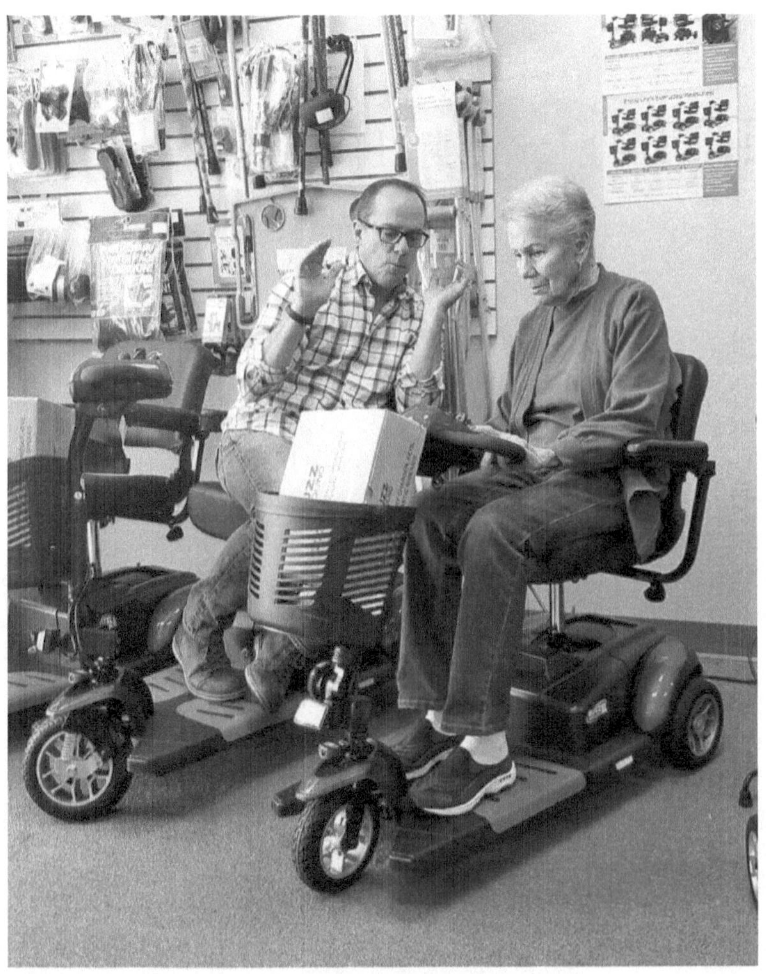

Mom testing the new scooter, which became known as
"The Beast".

CHAPTER 27

FRIENDS OF PARKINSON'S

IN MY SEARCH for support, I found an organization called Friends of Parkinson's located in West Las Vegas. They are a non-profit organization providing support and resources to Parkinson's patients and their families. Browsing through their website I learned they were holding a Wellness Symposium the following Saturday, focused on Medical Marijuana. The symposium was free of charge, but required registration, so I called their office and registered.

The following Saturday I drove across town to West Las Vegas. The Friends of Parkinson's organization was located in a small strip mall. I timidly opened the door to where I thought the meeting was being held and asked, "Is this where the Friends of Parkinson's is meeting?"

"You're in the right place," a friendly lady said, "Come on in. I'm assuming you have registered."

"Yes, I did," I said, feeling a bit more confident.

After I signed my name, I was invited to take a plate and add some snacks. I put some celery and carrots on my plate, along with some ranch dip and then helped myself to some cheese and crackers. They had created a very social setting. I helped myself to a bottle of water and wandered into a larger area set up as a classroom with rows of chairs all facing the front of the room. I chose to sit on the left side of the room, so my left-handed note taking didn't bother others. It also gave me a bird's eye view of the people entering the building. The others who joined the group were a varied mix of individuals.

The speaker stepped forward and introduced himself as a doctor and for two full hours, I took copious amounts of notes about marijuana and its effects on the brain. Marijuana and its THC properties can ease the muscle spasms and pain Parkinson's patients might experience. The question and answer session gave us a chance to hear personal stories and reasons for attending the symposium. Some of the participants were Parkinson's patients, while others were caregivers. Some, like myself, were family members wanting to learn more about the disease, and how medical marijuana could help the Parkinson's patient.

Once the class was finished, I was able to acquire a Medicinal Marijuana prescription, allowing me to purchase marijuana products ahead of the line at the Marijuana dispensary located right next door. It appeared to be a great little racket between the doctor, the dispensary and The Friends of Parkinson's. Each was gaining recognition.

Speaking with the doctor who presented the symposium, I asked, "How will the gummies affect me since I have had a double bypass and am taking blood pressure medication?"

"You will want to cut the gummies into ten small pieces, and take only one small portion to see how that small portion affects you," he said.

"What will happen?" I asked him, curious as to how my body would react.

"Your heart may race too fast, and it could make you feel very un-comfortable. You could even experience a heart attack." Participants may experience an increase in heart rate, dizziness, and impaired memory while using marijuana. "When you see how that one small piece affects you," he said, "you can decide to increase the dosage by taking two pieces the next day, but don't try it the same day," he warned.

"So one gummy could last me a long time," I laughed.

He chuckled at my statement. "That's true," he said, "but this should be done over a course of several days, while monitoring your heart rate. You'll also want to do the same technique with your eighty-five year old mother to see how she reacts to the THC."

"Thank you for your presentation," I said, "It was very enlightening." As I headed out the door, I felt a sense of euphoria come over me. I felt empowered with my new knowledge.

The dispensary next door to The Friends of Parkinson's office was a wall of glass. Outside the dispensary I saw a large sign that read, CASH ONLY. Never traveling with any cash, I gave up the idea of purchasing anything in the dispensary, but I wanted to take a look around. As I entered the glass door, a friendly lady welcomed me. She asked to see my driver's license. She appeared to be in her sixties, and was sitting on a stool in the small glass enclosure between the first glass door and the second glass door. There was barely enough room for the two of us to stand inside the glass cubicle, and I was relieved when the door opened and I was invited into the showroom.

Entering the showroom, I was greeted by a second elderly lady, sitting on another stool. This woman also requested to see my ID. Both ladies appeared to be of retirement age, and I immediately thought, "This would be a cool retirement position." To say the dispensary's security was tight would be an understatement. It was as if I had stepped into a James Bond film called <u>High Security for High Rollers</u>. Everything appeared to be high class and under lock and key. I was mesmerized by the sparkle and glitz in front of my eyes.

Bright lights illuminated glass cases that appeared to be floating against mirrored walls in this twenty by twenty square foot room. The shimmering lights reflected the glass receptacles surrounding the room like a jewelry store. Individual glass containers held marijuana products displayed one by one in each of the glass cases. Iridescent rainbows shimmered around the room as fragments of light bounced off the myriad of mirrors. There were glass islands strategically placed in the middle of the room, creating a type of maze one could meander around. Their metallic legs reflected the elegant radiance of the room. Instead of sparkling diamond rings and bracelets enclosed in the glass cases like a jewelry store, the boxes and bottles of marijuana products were highlighted in each individual case. I felt as if I were Audrey Hepburn in <u>Breakfast at Tiffany's</u>, but I certainly wasn't dressed for the glitz and glamor of this store. Everything sparkled.

As I shuffled my way through the line, my eyes were bouncing back and forth as if possessed by lasers. Scanning the customers, scanning the budtenders and the impressive products, I wanted to understand the procedures. As people made their way through the small sanctuary of cannabis, I noticed patrons showing their ID's again when making a selection with the budtender and again when they paid the cashier. I was overwhelmed with the security. My eyes gawked around the room when one of the budtenders asked, "Do you need any help?"

"Oh! No, thank you." I said, my eyes wide with wonder at what I was witnessing. "I'm just looking!" I stammered. She must have known I was a first timer. Embarrassed, I made my way to the exit, eager to share my newfound experience with Mom.

Returning to the car, glad to duck out of the rain, I sat down in the driver's seat. "Holy cow," I said to myself. "Now I know what to expect when I go into one of these dispensaries to get Mom some marijuana," I said to myself. I mentally made a note of the hours the store would be open, and the fact I would need lots of cash! Starting the car, adrenaline was coursing through my veins. It was as if I had just downed two cups of coffee. The excitement to share what I'd just seen was exhilarating. "I feel like I'm in another world," I said to myself. Everything around me felt strange. As if to accentuate that ominous feeling, the rain and dismal gray skies cast an eerie atmosphere over the area. It didn't feel like I was in Las Vegas any more. Everything felt bizarre.

Driving the forty-five minutes back to The Bridge, I was anxious to share the symposium information with Mom. I was sure she would be eager to try cannabis. I just knew she'd want to alleviate some of the tremors she'd been encountering inside her body. Knocking on her door, I rushed in, "It's me," I announced. "You're not going to believe this! Marijuana can help alleviate some of the symptoms of Parkinson's. It can ease the feeling of tremors and can make you feel better," I said, rambling on as fast as I could, almost dancing around Mom's room, grinning from ear to ear.

"No, thank you," Mom said, in her usual monotone voice as she looked down at her hands.

"What?" I said. "Marijuana is legal in Nevada, and I think it could help eliminate the tremors you're feeling inside your body," I said, giddy with excitement.

"No." she said. "I don't want to try it." She wouldn't even look at me! This was exasperating, and I couldn't contain my frustration.

"I just sat through a two hour class to get a medical certificate so I can purchase medicinal marijuana for you without having to stand in a long line, and you don't want to try it?" I asked, gasping for a breath as I blurted out my frustration. I was perplexed at Mom's answer.

"Nope," I don't want any," she stated bluntly. "Lann already sent me some drops, and I don't want to try them!"

"But they have chewable gummies. You don't have to smoke a joint anymore," I told her.

"No," she said, "I'm not going to try that stuff," she said adamantly. "I'm just not into it."

Case closed. Mom and I weren't going to get high together! She wanted nothing to do with marijuana or any of its products, and quite frankly, neither did I after learning what the THC could do to my heart condition. The doctor had explained to me I needed to be very careful, and it was at that point in time, I realized Mom also had a heart condition. Medical marijuana was not for us, but the entire day was an educational experience I'll never forget!

More education was on the way. A month later, the Friends of Parkinson's decided to hold their monthly meeting at The Bridge. That was exciting news to me, and I wanted Mom to meet the men and women in charge. They had been so friendly when I had visited their office for the symposium, and I wanted Mom to have a chance to meet other Parkinson's patients.

Wheeling her to lunch that day, I said, "The Friends of Parkinson's group is here for their monthly meeting. Let's go over and say hi."

"No, you can go if you want to," said Mom. She was embarrassed, afraid of having others look at her. She didn't want to be singled out at The Bridge as someone with Parkinson's. People were already talking about her being different. Although her tremors weren't visible, her choking spells brought her more attention than she cared to think about. When she wasn't in control of her body, she was ill equipped to deal with life around her.

"Don't you want to at least meet the leader?" I asked, nodding towards the living room area where guests were arriving.

"No, it's just not for me," she muttered. "You can go over there if you want to, but I don't want to." In true Mom fashion, she was not going to participate.

Although Mom didn't have visible shaking, tremors were internally ravaging her body, especially if she was nervous or cold. "You just don't know what it feels like to be inside my body," she said.

"You're right," I told her, not knowing exactly what else I could say.

"Well, I just hope you don't have to ever experience this," she said, reaching out to put her water bottle on the table in front of us. She had started carrying a miniature water bottle. She had determined the water at The Bridge was soft water, and the salt was making her legs swell up. Besides, a bottle of water was easier to handle than a glass of water.

"I hope so, too." I said. "I'm sure it's miserable." As I pushed her into her special dining room table, I could smell the sloppy joes. I knew they would serve the Friends of Parkinson's the same meal. "There's still plenty of time to go join the meeting," I said, "and you can get your lunch served over there."

"No," she said, "I can see them from here." A man was in our direct line of sight. He was hunched over; and his head was wobbling to and fro. Mom had a difficult time seeing someone with tremors. "I don't need to get any closer," she reiterated her desire to steer clear of the entire group.

"Okay," I said, "but I'm sure they would love to have us join them."

"You go, if you want to," Mom said again, "but I'm fine right here." It was as if she didn't want to join the leper colony, and it made me sad.

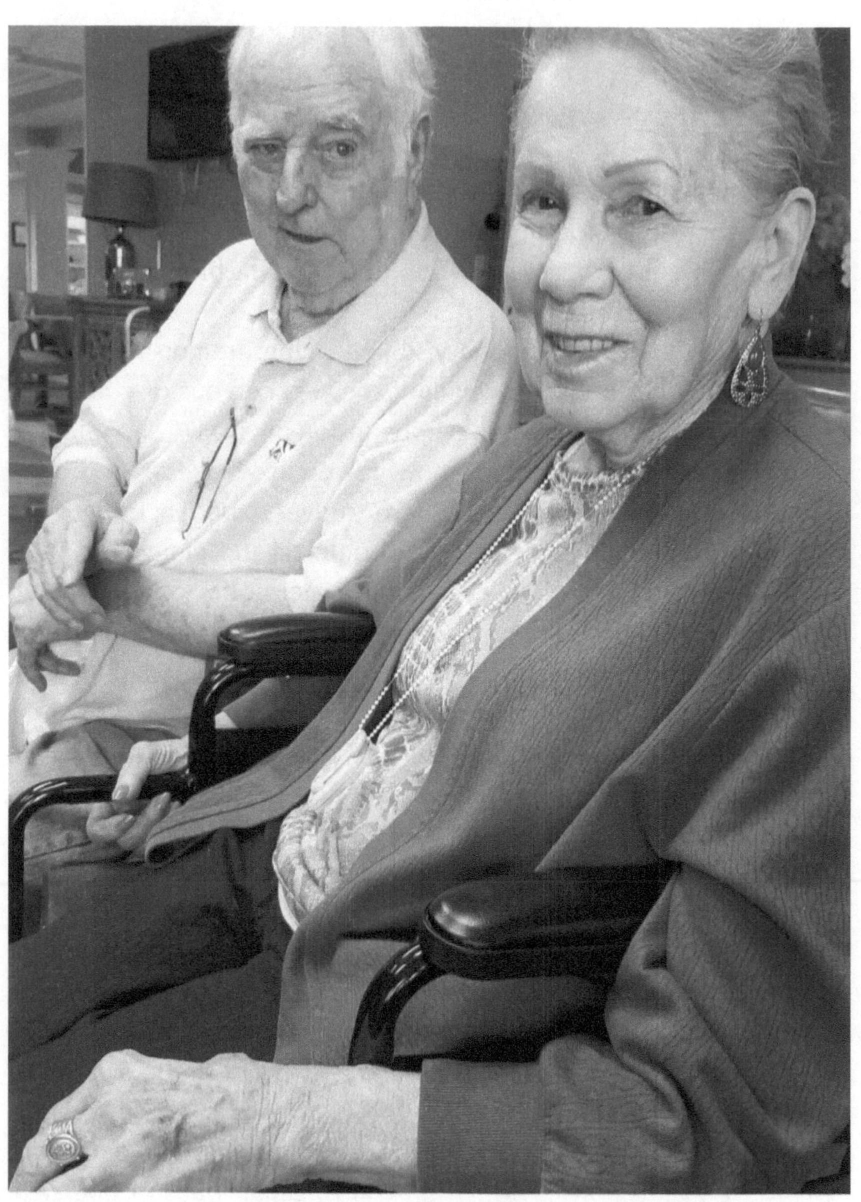

Mom with her friend, Owen

CHAPTER **28**

MEMORIES

SADNESS SEEMED TO surround us in our daily lives. I'd fly home and Mom would call with some kind of incident, and I would fly back. Trying to limit my time in Las Vegas to one week a month was not easy. Each visit brought different circumstances. So and so did this, or so and so did that. I learned to remember there were two sides of the story, just as I had to learn when my own children were reporting what had happened to them at school. Sometimes Mom's stories were a bit exaggerated.

Mom was a lover of reading, so she insisted her book sit on the end table near her chair as usual. But I often wondered just how much she was able to read, or absorb while she was trying to read. That book sat on her side table for the entire two years she was at The Bridge! I knew she could barely hold the large volume; and I didn't want to ask her about her eyesight.

She had several pairs of glasses stashed inside her nightstand, and one on top of her book. Her "readers", as she called them, were never far away. She used them to read her morning newspaper, but I wasn't sure just how much her eyesight had deteriorated. I didn't dare ask. Taking her to the eye doctor would be a fiasco. After all, we had stopped seeing her neurologist, and I didn't dare ask about an eye doctor or a dentist.

Knowing Mom enjoyed reading, I told her she might have fun

157

listening to books by using new technology. She had seen the Echo Dot being used in the main living area of the facility to play songs. "New technology is the way to go," I excitedly told Mom. She nodded.

We purchased an Echo Dot and set it up in her room. We practiced having Mom say, "Alexa, play my favorite song." Unfortunately, Mom's voice wasn't strong enough or clear enough to get the little machine to play songs or stories, so we gave up on the idea of having her listen to stories. Yelling at Alexa gave her a chance to practice her shouting voice, and every now and then she would get it to play her favorite song.

The Bridge offered several musical presentations, and I enjoyed these concerts immensely. They provided a nice break in the monotony of the afternoons. There was an Elvis impersonator who was quite good, along with several other performers. At first Mom didn't want to attend. She was concerned about what others would say about her. At eighty-five years old, she was still worried about what others were thinking. Eventually, with a little coaxing, I was able to get her to go along with me. I did have to tell her I was the one pushing the wheelchair, so she had to go where I pushed!

"I never did like Elvis Presley when I was younger," she said one day, her negative attitude shining through.

"Well, I want to hear this guy," I told her, "and since I'm pushing the wheelchair, I guess we'll just have to check him out." I knew Mom craved the socialization that these get-togethers offered. Also being musical, I knew she would enjoy herself once we were there. I had to learn to just ignore her dissension and take her to the performances. They certainly helped pass the long afternoons.

Eventually, a new activities director added even more activities, and Mom enjoyed the Wednesday afternoon wine social, along with the Bingo games. The new activities director also included games that required word knowledge and science knowledge. Mom became more interested in participating. These social activities not only helped the elderly residents, but they were paramount for the Parkinson's patients who try to isolate themselves. Like Mom, Parkinson's patients don't want to participate in social settings because they feel conspicuous.

Along with the wine tasting and concerts, Mom developed a little love interest in a gentleman named Owen, who started showing interest in her. With that interest, Mom started participating in more afternoon activities. It was even more exhilarating to have Owen come and eat lunch or dinner with us at Mom's table. His companionship was irreplaceable.

As a music teacher, I loved to watch the entertainers, but what was even more fun for me was entertaining the residents myself. A few evenings after dinner I would play the piano, and some of the residents would surround me and sing along. Sometimes I would just play music while they ate their evening meal, but I always enjoyed entertaining them.

Mom, Cathy, and I had often sung together when we were younger, and Mom was a wonderful musician who enjoyed hearing me sing. One evening, surrounded by the residents, I noticed that Mom had disappeared. Knowing she couldn't go anywhere on her own, I assumed she had called Cameron to take her to her room. "Maybe this little impromptu concert has thrown her out of her routine or maybe she needed to go back to use the bathroom," I thought, as I continued to play and sing.

A few minutes later, Cameron, her favorite CNA came and whispered in confidence, "Your Mom got too emotional this evening. She had me take her back to her room. You can take your time. There's no hurry."

It dawned on me, Mom was facing her mortality square in the eye. We didn't know how much longer she had. Listening to me sing the many songs we'd experienced together over the years was emotionally draining for her. I had sung songs from my wedding and many of the songs we shared through the years. I could tell Mom was probably wondering the same thing I was, "Is this the last time I will hear my daughter sing these songs?" I, too, became emotional.

Ending my little concert, I walked back to her room. "It's just me," I said as I walked into her room.

"I'm tired," Mom sighed, the Parkinson's fish face was more pronounced than ever.

"It's been a big day," I agreed, and the two of us sat in silence, watching a Hallmark movie. It wasn't anything either of us talked about, but emotions were very close to the surface that night. We both knew her time here on earth was nearing its end.

Mom had been in stage five for quite some time. We had read about the masked face or fish face. Parkinson's patients lose control of their facial muscles, they develop an open stare accompanied with an open mouth, similar to that of a fish with an open mouth. Mom dreaded this symptom, and only displayed the dreaded fish face late in her Parkinson's journey. Along with the drooling, Mom would have been mortified if I had told her she was exhibiting the fish face.

One thing we learned about Parkinson's is that everyone is on his/her own journey, and no two are alike. Symptoms are different for everyone, but when the fish face appeared, I recognized we were closer to the end of Mom's life.

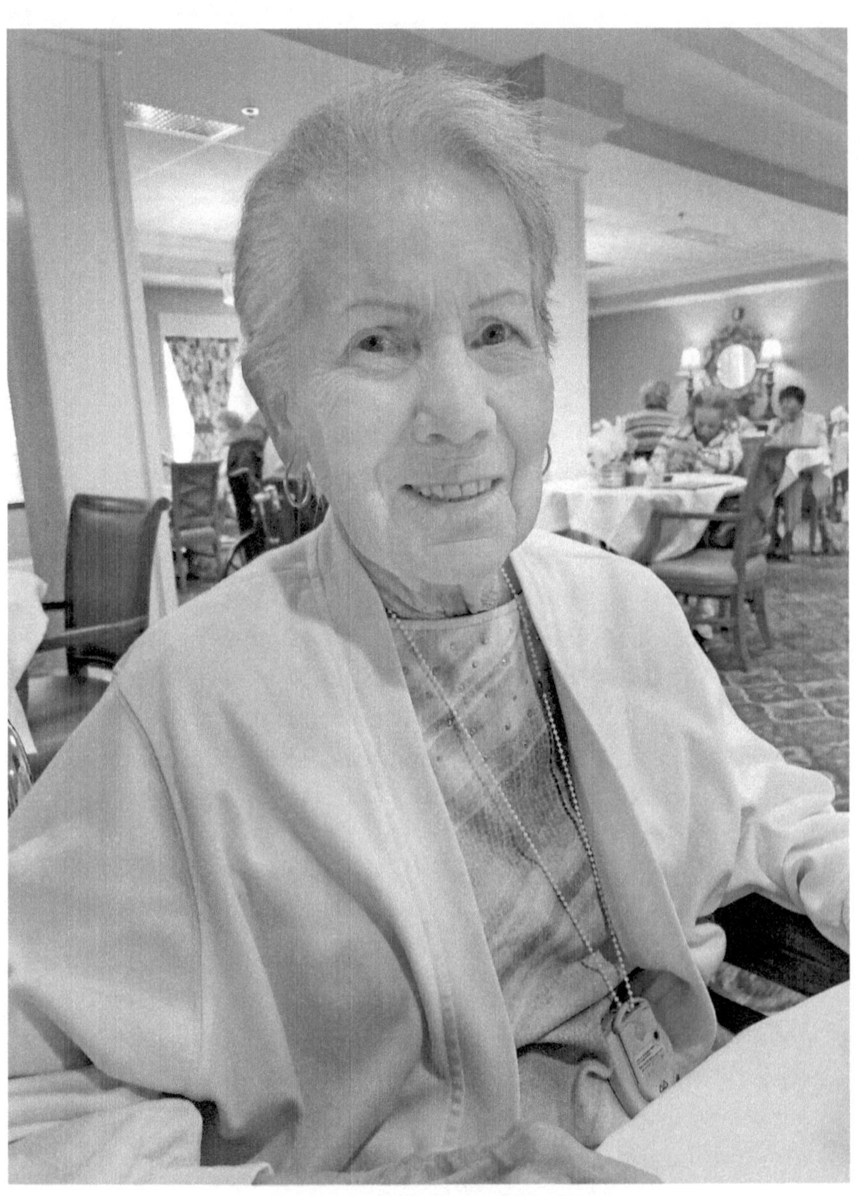

Mom in The Bridge dining room.

CHAPTER 29

PAPERWORK NECESSITIES

WHEN MOM WAS initially diagnosed with Parkinson's, I read some books. One book I read was called, <u>Old Parents and Purple Tulips;</u> <u>Navigating the Maze of Care-giving, Dementia, Sibling Conflict and</u> <u>Guns</u> by Betty Alder. Although Mom didn't have dementia, wasn't a hoarder, and didn't have any guns, I learned two major facts from this book. First, as the executor of Mom's estate, I needed to make sure I was on all her financial accounts; and second, I needed to be in charge of her medical directive. This would enable me to oversee what was happening financially and medically.

Long before Mom was diagnosed with Parkinson's, Cathy discovered Mom had been paying for two warranties on her car at the same time. Both warranties were being taken out of her bank account from the same company. We were also concerned that she was unnecessarily making purchases online. One company convinced her to pay a fifteen dollar monthly fee to enable her to receive a fifteen percent discount on her purchases. She wasn't making enough purchases to warrant this fifteen dollar a month fee, and we realized companies were taking advantage of her.

Another item showing up on her bank statement was a recurring charge of $19.99. After several telephone calls, I finally discovered some company was swindling her out of twenty dollars a month, and she had no idea who or why. Fortunately, the bank verified this as a fraudulent charge, telling me many seniors were being taken advantage of through this scheme. They were able to reimburse those fraudulent charges.

With this premise in mind, Mom and I went to the bank. We wanted to put my name on her accounts, thus allowing me to oversee her expenditures. I explained to the manager at the bank, "I want to have my name added to my Mom's accounts."

"She's my daughter," Mom said, "and she is the executor of my estate," Mom explained to the manager.

"You're already listed as the executor for your mother's estate, so you don't need to have your name on her bank accounts," the manager told us. She was a stern looking lady, dressed in a business suit. "When your mother passes away, you will deal with her accounts, but until then, you don't need to be on the accounts." She obviously didn't understand my desire to be a co-signer on the accounts. I wanted to be able to sign checks on Mom's account and keep an eye on what was happening. I didn't have the heart to explain my true desire in front of Mom, not wanting to upset her or hurt her feelings. After all, Mom had been in control of the family's finances for fifty years. I knew as the executor, I would indeed handle the account when Mom passed away.

"All you have to do when your Mom passes away is bring a copy of the death certificate to the bank, and we will help you at that time," stated the bank manager.

Not wanting to show my frustration, Mom and I politely completed our other transactions and left. In hindsight, I should have taken the grumpy looking bank manager aside and explained what was happening, but at the time, Mom looked like a whipped puppy. I knew her feelings were very fragile, so I acquiesced.

The bright side of this incident was that with Mom's help, I was able to access her bank account by setting up an online account. In today's world, I know that sounds absurd, but at the time, it was a unique situation for Mom. Our dilemma was solved. I could easily keep an eye on Mom's account. My advice for anyone with an elderly family member would be to obtain access to their finances; so no one can obtain access to those funds until after probate.

Mom was fortunate. Her husband had established a Family Trust years earlier. This meant Mom became the director of the Family Trust upon his passing. It also meant in the state of Nevada, the Family Trust didn't have to go through probate. Mom felt it was necessary to keep the Family Trust up to date, so she spent quite a bit of money at the attorney's office ensuring her daughters' name changes were listed correctly. One daughter remarried; and one daughter legally changed her name. So Mom paid to have those corrections made to the Trust. She also felt she was no longer capable of carrying out the Trust directives. Therefore, she again paid her attorney to list my husband and me as the directors of the Trust. Even though we were already listed as the executors, she wanted us to be listed as the directors of the funds, in case she was unable to fulfill any duties prior to her death.

Definitely proactive about her estate, Mom's last will and testament were included in the Family Trust. She made sure David and I understood what the will said, and where it was located. She gave me her attorney's name and where he was located, and David and I visited his office when we signed the paperwork to become the Directors of the Estate.

The second thing I learned from the book, <u>Old People and Purple Tulips</u>, was to designate one person to be the health director. This is the one, and only person, medical personnel are allowed to contact for any, and all, medical decisions. The person designated as the medical director doesn't have to be the same person as the executor. In fact, it might be better to have two people working together; one working with the Parkinson's patient's health, and one in charge of the financial documents. One thing was clear, it is paramount that only one person be in charge of the advanced directive. This ensures no cross communication. The health care directive should state the patient's desires; and the health care director should be confident in carrying out those wishes.

In the above mentioned book, Betty Alder waited too long to

process these documents. Her parents did not have an advanced directive or Living Will, and she was not able to be in charge of their medical care. She did not have a power of attorney, and therefore could not handle any of the financial needs. By the time Betty needed these documents in place, her parents were not of sound mind to make the decisions, and Betty had to take legal action to become a legal guardian for her parents. Going through the court system was a painful process for her as well as her parents, who didn't understand what was happening.

We were lucky Mom had everything in order and worked within the Family Trust. It made my job as the medical director and financial director a breeze. As executors, David and I were able to complete the distribution of assets within a few months of her passing, amazing family at how efficiently we were able to carry out Mom's wishes. It was all due to her proper planning.

Looking back, I wish I had done more research on the care of elderly family members, but this book gave David and me the impetus to make sure our own documentation is now in place. As you face this stage of life with your parents and loved ones, I highly recommend you seek out as much information as you can handle.

In planning ahead, Mom had purchased long term care insurance. It was to provide her with assistance when she couldn't care for herself with daily living, such as eating, bathing and dressing. Unfortunately, Mom felt she was unable to continue paying for this insurance, and canceled it. It could have been quite beneficial while she was living in The Bridge. If you can afford long term care, it is very beneficial.

We were not full time caregivers, but instead, we were overseers of Mom's care. Years earlier, Mom had made it quite clear she didn't want us interrupting our lives to care for her. "I watched your father's family take care of their mothers and fathers, and they couldn't go anywhere or do anything. I don't want you to do that for me," she had said.

Mom's philosophy allowed me to travel as a snowbird and still visit her when needed. At times I was located fifteen hours away, and at other times only five hours away. I was thankful to be able to continue my own activities.

If you find yourself faced with being a full time caregiver, please find someone to join you in that task. I was fortunate to have my sister, Cathy, join me in Mom's care. We tried to alternate our visits, sharing in the responsibility, but in the end, I was the person solely responsible.

If you are raising your own children while caring for your parents, please ask for help. Being part of the sandwich generation is a challenge. It is enough work to raise your own children, but to care for your parents at the same time is highly stressful. Seek out other family members or members from a church to help take up some of the slack in caring for your parents. Retirement homes and assisted living facilities are wonderful, but a family member still needs to oversee the care they provide. Stay in touch with those facilities on a weekly basis.

When Mom initially downsized and moved into the retirement home, she decided to obtain a DNR. This stands for Do Not Resuscitate. "Don't let anyone come in here and pound on my chest to bring me back to life," she said. "Just let me die a natural death."

"So, you don't want any CPR?" I asked, reiterating what Mom wanted.

"No, I don't want any extreme measures to keep me alive," she said, "Just let me go. If it's my time, it's my time," she added, her voice more slurred from Parkinson's.

"No hospital- No ambulances- I got it," I said. "Anything else I should know?" I asked.

"Just let me die a natural death with no bells and whistles. You can celebrate later," she said with a smile on her face.

"No bells and whistles," I laughed, as I waved my hand in a circular motion above my head. We both giggled. "Oh, we'll celebrate," I said. "You can bet your sweet bippy, we'll celebrate!" and the two of us laughed even harder.

I understood what Mom meant. She didn't want to be tube fed. She didn't want dialysis. She didn't want oxygen, and she definitely didn't want anybody pounding on her chest. I placed the paperwork on the refrigerator of her retirement home, the bright red DNR showing prominently through the plastic envelope. Behind the DNR was Mom's advanced health directive. "Now the paramedics should see your DNR when they come in to help you, but I doubt it's going to be anytime soon." I said.

At the next doctor's appointment, Mom's doctor suggested I obtain a medical power of attorney.

"But I have a regular Power of Attorney," I told her doctor.

"The more documentation, the better," he said, "You just never know."

"I have a Power of Attorney," I said, "and I am the director of her Advanced Medical Directive, and I am one of the directors of her Irrevocable Trust, and you still want me to get a Medical power of attorney?" I asked.

"That's right," said the doctor. You'll have all of your bases covered in case anyone questions the decisions you make. You can't be too careful these days," he said. "You know relatives!"

"I get it," I said, looking at Mom. "Now, no one will question what you want and what I have done," I told her. "You want to have a natural death, so we have the DNR in place, and I know where the will, the trust, the advanced health directive and the two powers of attorney are located. I think we have everything in place. What else do you want?" I asked Mom.

"I put all of the instructions for my funeral in the metal box with all of the other paperwork," she said. "It should be easy to find. By the way, where is that metal box?" she asked for the thousandth time!

"It's in the closet," I told her. "Since we're on the subject, tell me some of the things you want at your funeral," I said. I was glad she was always willing to discuss her passing with me.

"I'm glad you want to talk about this," she said, "Cathy never wants to discuss my dying. I think she is going to have a difficult time with it when it happens."

"Well, I want to be sure to do what you want," I assured her, walking over to the closet to pull out the metal box. Sliding the heavy gray box across the floor, I maneuvered so it sat in front of my chair. I opened it.

"There it is," Mom said, excitedly watching me steer the precious metal box across the floor. "It's got everything in there."

"Yes," I said, "we look at it every time I visit you."

"I want a bagpiper to play during the service," she said. "There's a paper in the box with a bagpiper's name. And I want Henry Snead to sing "His Eye is On the Sparrow", she said.

"How do I get in touch with Henry? What was his last name again?" I asked, perplexed at never hearing this man's name before. It was as if my mother had a life I didn't know about!

"Snead," she said. "It rhymes with shed. Just check with the minister, she'll be able to give you Henry's number. I'd like to have him play a bunch of gospel songs before or during the service. They always make me happy," she said.

"That sounds easy enough," I said. "Do you want the funeral at the church or at the mortuary where we had Doc's memorial?" I asked her.

"Oh, I'd like it to be at the church," she told me, "I didn't keep paying my tithe for nothing. I was just paying for my funeral in advance!" We both giggled. She was definitely planning ahead.

"You can get the minister's number out of my address book," she said, reaching for her little red address book in her night stand. "You can call my friend, Gail, she's in charge of putting on the receptions after the funerals. She'll do a nice job of decorating for you."

"Wow, you've got this all organized," And then using my best southern accent I added, "We're definitely going to celebrate!".

"Well," she said, "I don't have much else to think about these days!" she smiled. "After Bill died, I marched Earl up to the mortuary with me, and I paid for my own funeral. I didn't want you girls to have to go through what I went through trying to figure everything out when you are so distraught. This way everything is paid for," she told me.

"That's pretty cool," I said, not knowing what else to say as I leafed through her little red address book.

"Everything you need should be in that metal box," she said. We spent some time leafing through the paperwork, but I didn't see anything specific regarding her memorial service. I'm glad she told me what she wanted.

I picked up the heavy container, and hefted it back to the closet. I must have told Mom where that metal box was stored every time I visited, but she was becoming more and more forgetful. Fortunately, she had her paperwork in order, and when I went home, I was happy to tell David, "Mom has everything in order for her last will and testament as well as her memorial service. I think we need to do the same thing."

David repeated a phrase he had learned in the navy, "Proper planning prevents piss-poor performance," he said. "So I guess we should get our wills and medical directives in order, too."

I can't stress enough how much easier this made Mom's passing for both of us, and I encourage everyone to get these documents in order. Your children will thank you! Thank you, Mom!

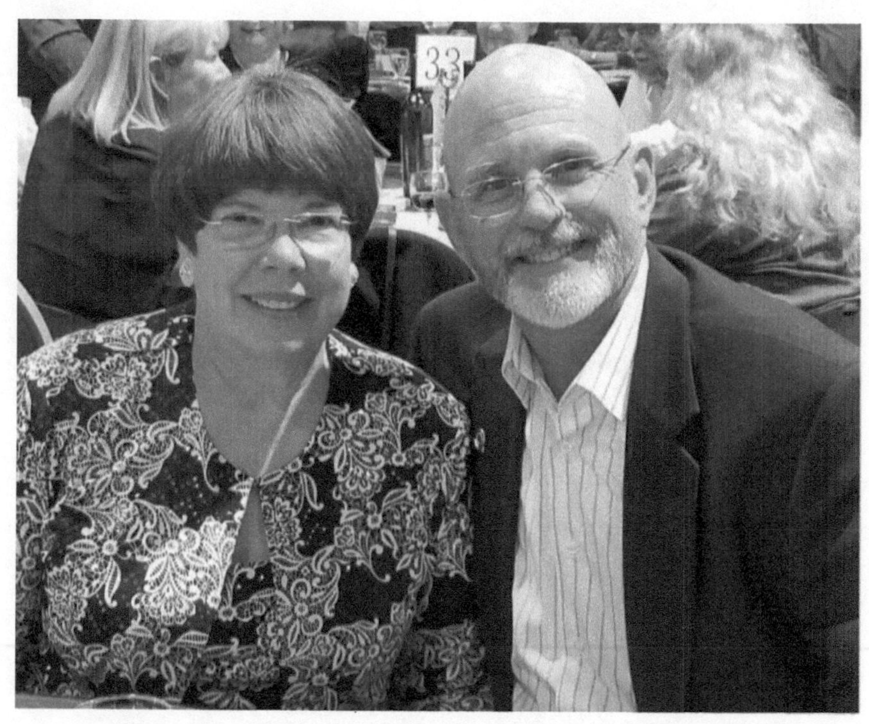

Caryn and David Mears, executor's of mom's Family Trust Fund.

CHAPTER 30

WHAT CAN WE DO NOW?

NOW THAT YOU have your last will and testament in order; along with your memorial service wishes and desires, it's time to look at the future of Parkinson's. Further research brought me to this statement from a review article produced March 4, 2022, called "Inflammation and Immune Dysfunction in Parkinson's Disease." It said, "Parkinson's is now understood to be a multi-system disorder with neuro-inflammation and immune dysfunction that has been implicated in the development of various non-motor symptoms such as sleep and gastrointestinal dysfunction, which can precede the disease diagnosis by decades." Phew! That was a ton to process! This enormously technical statement basically says sleep studies and gastrointestinal evaluations have been able to recognize Parkinson's disease decades in advance of the actual diagnosis.

We joke about being stiff in the morning and slow to get moving; and we joke about poor sleep and forgetfulness. We attribute all these symptoms to growing old. However, for Parkinson's patients these symptoms are no joke. They are symptoms they face every day. Kathleen Washalup from the Oxford Parkinson's Disease Centre Cohort stated "As our population ages, we are becoming more prone to Parkinson's." Some of the research concentrates on sleep disorders and REM Behavior Disorder. Recognizing patients with these two sleep disorders has led to the discovery that Parkinson's patients who have problems with memory function, mood disorders, daytime sleepiness and anxiety, have had REM Behavior Disorder well before being diagnosed with Parkinson's.

The Oxford Parkinson's Disease Centre also discovered that cognitive differences and memory changes factor into Parkinson's diagnosis with early signs of apathy, pain, fatigue, and depression, and forgetfulness. These developments were also noted in the physiological motor symptoms with changes in speech, tremors, stiffness, and balance.

Another article written by Steve Peterson called "I Used to Suffer Parkinson's" encourages Parkinson's patients to try the Parkinson's Protocol. In a walking advertisement for the Parkinson's Protocol, Peterson discusses the hows and whys of Parkinson's, and goes on to explain some things patients can do to help eliminate symptoms. There is worthwhile information in the article, even if you don't want to pay for the protocol. It appears to be very beneficial if you are diagnosed early in life. The average age for a Parkinson's diagnosis is sixty-five, while Michael J. Fox was diagnosed at the age of twenty-nine.

Parkinson's is an illness caused by loss of the body's ability to produce dopamine. So why do some people get Parkinson's while others do not? This is the million dollar question science is trying to answer. Many researchers believe there are two causes; one is genetic while the other is environmental toxins.

The first question most people have upon diagnosis is, "Why me?", followed by "Will my children inherit this disease?" However, the most pronounced question of all is "How did I get Parkinson's?"

Dopamine is the chemical in the brain that controls movement, memory, pleasurable rewards, and motivation. It is being depleted, and this loss of dopamine is associated with several mental health and neurological diseases, one of which is Parkinson's. You and I are both asking, "How can we increase our dopamine levels?" One way is to avoid overindulging in alcohol or recreational drug use. Although we think of these as "feel good supplements", they are actually depressants. So one of the first things to do is to stop alcohol consumption.

We can also increase dopamine levels by eating a healthy diet. A diet high in magnesium, including nuts, spinach, tuna, and scallops along with white and black beans will help. Tyrosine will as well. It can be found in chicken, turkey, fish, peanuts, almonds, avocados, bananas, milk, cheese, yogurt, cottage cheese, lima beans, pumpkin seeds, and sesame seeds. A diet high in these two compounds appears to increase dopamine levels. However, before you think, "I could just take extra magnesium and tyrosine supplements," please check with your doctor. These supplements have the ability to negatively interact with other medications, and create negative side effects.

Eating a healthy diet means we're avoiding junk food, right? Junk food is very detrimental to increasing dopamine. Although it makes us feel better for a short time, it is detrimental to increasing dopamine. So, give up junk food too!

An activity that increases dopamine is exercise. It is a beneficial activity no matter what ails you. Plus, exercise is free! Being outside also increases dopamine levels, so if you exercise outdoors, you are actually increasing your dopamine levels in two ways. Studies show that just walking thirty minutes a day is beneficial for cardio health, bone health, and muscle health. Personally, I break thirty minute walks into two fifteen minute segments. It's an easy way to increase dopamine levels in your brain, and who knows, maybe while you're walking, you'll keep going a little longer!

A good sleep routine is another recommendation to increase dopamine levels, along with practicing meditation or yoga. All of these activities help our body feel good, which in turn increases our dopamine levels. If you are struggling with sleep, consult a doctor. Sleep disorders and slight tremors are the first symptoms Parkinson's patients experience.

Mom smoked for fifty years, so I often ask myself, "Was smoking the toxin that caused Mom's dopamine levels to drop?" Next I ask myself, "If Mom hadn't smoked in twenty five years, was it just old age that brought on Parkinson's?" She wasn't diagnosed until she was eighty-four, but I'm sure she had the symptoms for several years prior to her diagnosis. As her daughter, like other Parkinson's sons and daughters, I worry whether I'm genetically predisposed to the disease. I tell myself, "Working towards a healthier lifestyle can't hurt."

It's not clear if Parkinson's is caused by environmental factors or genetics. About ten to fifteen percent of all Parkinson's is genetically related. A handful of ethnic groups, such as the Ashkenazi Jews from the Rhineland of Germany, and the North African Arab Barbers located on the Mediterranean Sea, have a higher propensity to carrying a mutational gene for Parkinson's, but it is not known why this gene is inherited. There are studies working on this question.

Even though Mom's neurologist told her that there are no medications that would help her type of Parkinson's, there are several different types of medications that treat Parkinson's symptoms. There are drugs to treat depression; drugs to treat tremors; drugs to treat cognition; and drugs to treat drooling. Levodopa is the most common drug on the market for raising dopamine levels, but a new drug called Fibroblast Growth Factor1 is being researched. It works by growing new blood vessels in the brain. In the next few years there will be several more drugs available to Parkinson's patients, so it is essential that you discuss this with your doctor.

Shortly after Mom's diagnosis, I received a phone call asking if Mom would be a good candidate for Deep Brain Stimulation. This is a surgical procedure for Parkinson's patients which helps to ease motor symptoms and decrease medication needs for some people. Since Mom was eighty-four years old when she was diagnosed, and did not do well in the hospital or the skilled nursing facility, I felt it wasn't in her best interest to expose her to a hospital situation again. She did not have major tremors and was not taking any medication, so I told them I didn't believe Mom was a good candidate for Deep Brain Stimulation. This is something you would need to discuss with your doctor. Many other Parkinson's patients have found it to be beneficial.

What Mom's doctor did suggest were therapists. A physical therapist can guide you through the right moves to increase mobility, such as working on side to side movements like swinging your arms while you walk. They may suggest a recumbent bicycle or elliptical machine to help practice these motor skills. They may also have chants or songs to help their patients continue a forward motion. Being a music teacher, I often tried to sing marching songs to get Mom to walk with a left-right progression, in order to help her through her freezing episodes. Unfortunately, Mom ended up in a wheelchair sooner than we expected, so this technique wasn't used long.

Physical therapists also share activities which enhance a Parkinson's patient's sense of strength and balance. These activities are meant to alleviate stiffness in the hip flexors, hamstrings and calf muscles by providing stretching while using resistance bands and light weights. The therapist usually shows the patient how to do these exercises in a safe manner when he/she isn't available, and it's best to practice these exercises several times a day, instead of once a day or once a week when the therapist visits. These strength training exercises are very beneficial to the Parkinson's patient gaining core strength which is important to walking independently.

As the disease progresses, occupational therapists can help Parkinson's patients stay active in their daily life by improving their fine motor skills. They will develop activities which address arm and hand movements, to aid in daily personal hygiene activities such as brushing teeth, combing hair and eating. Occupational therapists can also identify equipment to help Parkinson's patients adapt to those activities. They show the Parkinson's patient new ways to dress themselves and toilet themselves. Basically they try to enhance the daily life of a Parkinson's patient.

Research shows that eighty-nine percent of Parkinson's patients experience speech and voice disorders. Their voices grow soft, or monotone, and lack articulation. As a result, they lose confidence to participate in conversations, and often feel isolated. Not only do Parkinson's patients experience stiffness in their extremities, they experience stiffness in their throat muscles. A speech therapist can implement techniques to increase voice volume, and help articulation, allowing Parkinson's patients to speak more clearly. They also address swallowing techniques since Parkinson's patients are also prone to choking. If you experience any vocal or swallowing changes, please request a referral from your physician for a speech therapist.

Inflammation is a prime cause of many diseases, and Parkinson's patients are no exception to inflammation. Some people feel that environmental toxins play a part in the onset of Parkinson's. Today, toxins, which are poisons to our bodies, are everywhere in our daily living. We face toxins from household furnishings, paints, toys, cleaning supplies, plastics, water, and even in the air we breathe. The build up of these toxins is becoming detrimental to our bodies. As our bodies break down these toxins, it is believed that toxins are causing degenerative brain diseases. The worst of which is Parkinson's. As a young girl, Mom would walk with her father through the fields spraying pesticides over the crops, and we find ourselves wondering if this toxin could be one of the main culprits for Mom's Parkinson's.

Mental stress is also debilitating, causing low moods, which can lower our dopamine levels. With the lower dopamine levels, comes lower levels of one's feelings of well-being. People who have been diagnosed with Parkinson's often feel depressed. It becomes a vicious cycle. When someone feels so depressed they can't even get up in the morning, it is unlikely they will be able to maintain a healthy lifestyle. They need people around them to encourage and care for them. One of the most important factors in a healthy lifestyle is maintaining good relationships. Find friends who aren't frightened by your Parkinson's diagnosis.

With cases of Parkinson's doubling over the past twenty-five years, we should realize something is causing this drastic upsurge of brain degeneration. Whether it is the environmental toxins, the changes in diet, or the isolation of our society, we need to realize we must tackle this as a society. We've been taught to take a drug to cure us or have an operation to fix us, but in actuality, lifestyle changes are what are going to make the biggest difference.

Jody Knapp from the Parkinson's Protocol states, "Diseases don't just happen. There are reasons we have ailments, and learning about the causes creating those ailments enables us to make the adjustments to turn our lives around." We have to learn why brain cells are dying, and we have to address the low dopamine levels, and then we can address the other symptoms of the disease.

At the Oxford Parkinson's Disease Centre, cutting edge technology is on the horizon. An Android wearable wristband is being tested to monitor balance, gait, manual dexterity and tremors during a three minute test. Dr. Max Little is also working on an Android app to distinguish voice progression and its changes. This research is bringing new technology to the forefront.

Calvin Close, a Parkinson patient from England, posted a video about his experience with HBOT therapy. According to Mr. Close, the Hyperbaric Oxygen Therapy has completely turned his Parkinson's around. At only fifty years of age, Close was one of the younger patients experiencing tremors in his arms, closed fists, the Parkinson's shuffle, and loss of smell. After his therapy, his hands were able to type again; he was able to walk without shuffling; and his sense of smell was returning. This may be something others will want to experiment with since Close has had such positive results. Again, check with your doctor!

I'd be remiss if I didn't mention The Michael J. Fox Foundation, where research teams are working diligently to recruit case study participants. Their relentless pursuit of better treatments, cures and disease prevention is to be commended. Imagine a scan that could reveal what is happening inside our brains, allowing doctors to make better diagnoses and scientists to understand if potential therapies are effective. I encourage you to sign up for The Michael J Fox Foundation Newsletter as well as the American Parkinson's Association Newsletter. Both entities have a wealth of information.

Looking back, Mom tried to live a healthy lifestyle. Unfortunately the damage had already been done by the time she received her Parkinson's diagnosis. That's when we wanted a drug to fix it, and the doctor told us there were no drugs for her type of Parkinson's. That's when we wanted surgery to fix it, and we realized surgery wasn't an option. That's when we were told, "Parkinson's is not completely diagnosed until they do an autopsy." However, for the thousands of Parkinson's patients, please understand your diagnosis by a neurologist is verifiable. Your shuffling and festinating gait, your tremors, and your soft speech qualify you for treatments. Your diagnosis is valid long before you are on the autopsy table.

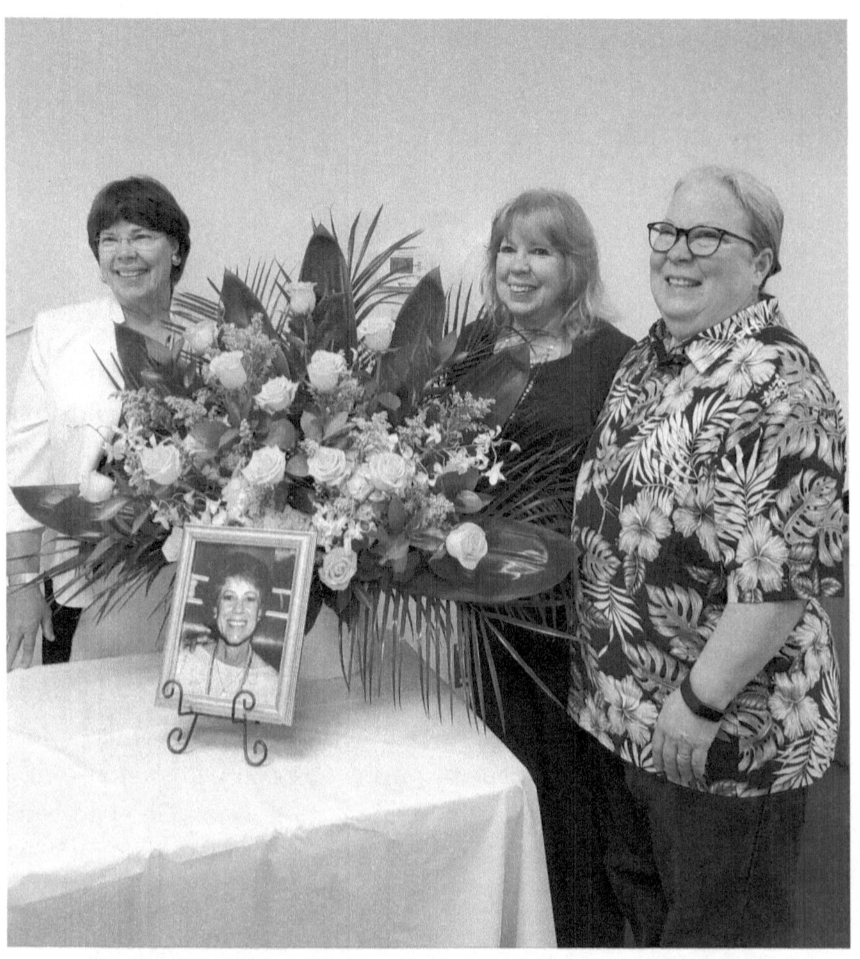

Mom's memorial service, March 12, 2020, with her three daughters; Caryn Mears, Cathy Peterson, and Lann Wilder.

CHAPTER 31

IT'S TIME

MY HOPE IN writing this book is to enlighten those who are facing this new journey; so when you hear your doctor say, "It's Parkinson's," you will be able to face the diagnosis with less fear and trepidation. Each of us has a different journey, but hopefully this book will make your Parkinson's journey easier.

During my last visit to Las Vegas in February of 2020, Mom was quite animated. Over the course of several afternoons, I finished reading the manuscript of the book she had started writing about her life. She had wanted to honor Alfred E. Bates, the man who adopted and raised her, by telling her story. She had gone on to raise three children of her own, become Mrs. Minnesota, and play in the Sands Hotel's orchestra in Las Vegas. When she was diagnosed with Parkinson's, I asked her if I could take over the writing of her book. She had been excited to share her unique story. "Oh that would be wonderful," she said, "I just can't do it anymore."

Opening the folder she had given me, I discovered Mom's notes looked like chicken scratching. The first portion of the manuscript had been typed by Cathy during her visits, but I ended up adding over twenty more chapters. Mom had only written about her growing up years and had just reached the first year of her marriage where I was born. Luckily, I still had Mom around, and she was more than willing to answer any questions I had about the writing of her biography.

Laying the manuscript of <u>Together Always</u> on the bed, I said, "Now I have to find a publisher, and then we'll actually see a real book."

Mom looked at me and asked, "Are you trying to finish this before I die?"

I looked her in the eye and laughed. "No! I'm trying to finish it before I die! You just never know," I chuckled, "you might outlast me!"

She seemed to ponder what I had just said. "You're going to get rich with this book," she said, as she looked straight at me. "It's so well done."

I laughed again. Getting up from my chair, I turned her wheelchair away from the bed. "I doubt that," I told her, "you just like this story because it's about you!"

"Well, I do think it's a pretty darn good story, if I do say so myself," she said.

"It is a wonderful story about a wonderful person," I told her. She smiled. "Let's head down to the science activity," I said, "it's something new the activities director has started."

Pushing Mom's wheelchair down the hall, we turned into the activities area, and nestled ourselves into the middle of the small group. Five or six other residents were there ready to be entertained with a science lesson. "Today's lesson is about tornadoes," said the activities director. Mom and I looked at each other with a sense of knowing. Mom had lived through a tornado as a young girl. She remembered the roar of the train as it passed overhead. She remembered the utter darkness when all of the electricity had been knocked out. She remembered the sound of building crumpling and cars being thrown down the street. She had kept a scrapbook of every newspaper article written about it. She also had many photographs her father had taken. This was a topic she knew well. It was right up her alley.

Throughout the presentation and discussion, Mom interjected information. She was very animated, and I almost felt like I had my old mom back. Afterwards, we stayed for a small glass of wine. Actually, I had my glass, as well as Mom's glass. She had quietly passed her glass to me, content to watch the others. Her friend, Owen, joined us, which brought a coy smile to her face.

Later that evening, after we had eaten dinner, we went back to Mom's room to watch the news, followed by a Hallmark movie. I was massaging Mom's legs with the special lotion, watching the fluid travel back up her leg. "I hope I'm not sending all of this fluid up to your heart," I said, and then added, "What if all that fluid kills you?"

"So be it," said Mom, "but I don't think I'll be that lucky."

"Now don't talk like that," I told her. "I'll be back at the end of the month, and Cathy is coming in March. She always has something she needs to shop for."

I put the massage towel and lotion back in the bathroom, and sat down in the green chair next to Mom. We both understood I would be leaving the next morning, so our emotions were running close to the surface. Leaving was always bittersweet for me. I looked forward to getting back home; but I was sad to leave Mom alone. We both had tears in our eyes as I bent over the top of her to give her a goodbye hug. "It's always so awkward trying to hug you in this chair," I said.

Mom replied, "I love you."

"I love you, too," I said, and then I scurried around the corner of her room and out the door, trying to keep from sobbing. Tears were welling up in my eyes, and I wanted to escape before they started to fall.

Once I was in the car, I heaved a huge sigh of relief. I hadn't cried in front of Mom. Reaching into my pocket, I discovered Mom's keys. Not wanting to go back into the building and go through another goodbye session, I decided I would drop them off early the next morning before I drove out of town.

The next morning, I stopped at The Bridge and rang the doorbell. A new aide opened the door, and I blurted, "Would you please put these keys in the pocket of my Mom's wheelchair?"

"Sure," said the aide.

I hurried back to my car, and started pulling out of the parking spot when it dawned on me that I hadn't told the new aide who my Mom was! "Oh well," I thought, "hopefully, her room number is on the key." Pushing the ignition, I was off on my five hour journey back to our winter home in Southern California. As I drove, I reminisced about the week I had just experienced. One of the aides had accidentally dropped Mom in the bathroom. Mom had hit her head on the floor, which prompted my visit. Number one, I needed to check on Mom and number two, I needed to let The Bridge staff know I was always aware of what was happening behind closed doors.

As I left the San Bernardino area, four hours into my journey, I received a call from the nurse at The Bridge. "Your Mother passed away early this morning," she said.

"You're kidding!" I exclaimed, thinking I had just been with her yesterday, and she was very animated.

"I wouldn't joke about something like this," said the voice on the other end of the phone. "Your Mom didn't want to get up this morning, so we let her sleep, and she passed away very peacefully. The doctor has signed her death certificate and her body will be taken to Palm Mortuary per your request."

"Thank you," I said. "I'll be back next week to clean out her room." I was dazed, but not wanting to turn around and drive four hours back to Las Vegas, I started calling those who needed to know Mom had passed. Secretly, I was wishing I had been there for Mom, but she had died on her own terms; no bells or whistles were involved.

Telling Cathy, made me choke up as my voice wavered, "Mom passed away this morning."

"Well, I'll never look at Valentine's Day the same," said Cathy, "I think Bill came down and swooped her up for a Valentine's dance in heaven." The day was February 14, 2020.

"That's a wonderful way to look at it," I said. "I had just asked Mom how people remember the day their loved ones pass. I guess she made sure I'd remember the date. I'll be going back next week to clean out her room," I told Cathy.

"I'll change my ticket so I can come and help you," she said, as we made plans to take care of Mom's possessions.

Mom died at the age of eighty-six years old, having lived a long, interesting life. Although she was diagnosed with Parkinson's at the age of eighty-four, we believe she probably was in the first stage when the family had descended upon her for her eightieth birthday celebration. She loved that attention, and now, planning her memorial service, we were going to be lavishing her with even more attention.

Mom's memorial took place on March 12, 2020, at the University Methodist Church in Las Vegas. She had been cremated and I had supplied the special box for her ashes, so I was surprised to see a hearse in the main parking lot when I pulled up to the church. The funeral director greeted me when I walked inside. "I have your Mother's ashes, and I'll place this beautiful box in the middle of the altar, if that's okay with you." he said.

"That's fabulous," I replied, "Mom always liked to be the center of attention." I said. "Why is the hearse here?" I asked.

"Your Mother paid for our services, and we thought the least we could do was bring her to her own memorial service in style," he answered.

"That's awesome," I said. "She would have liked that."

All three daughters spoke at the memorial service, as did one grandson-in-law whom Mom had chosen. He was married to her oldest granddaughter, Carissa, and he spoke of how supportive Mom had been during their courtship and marriage. Six of her seven grandchildren were able to be at the service, even though they were spread around the nation. My oldest daughter, Mollie, was not able to attend since she was stationed in Japan.

The bagpiper played "Amazing Grace," and Henry Snead sang, "His Eye is on the Sparrow." I was enthralled, and completely understood why Mom had chosen Henry to sing. His long dreadlocks reminded me of Ray Charles, as he swayed to the music he played on the piano. His voice was soulful, melodic, and powerful. The organist played several spirituals as the family gathered together to pay tribute to this phenomenal woman. The female minister delivered a wonderful eulogy; and I found myself smiling during the entire service, knowing Mom would be happy with her service

Coming out of the church, I discovered the hearse was still parked in the parking lot. "What are you still doing here," I asked the funeral director.

"The hearse won't start," he said. "I think the battery's dead, so I'm having someone come and jump it."

I laughed, "Mom would have gotten a chuckle out of this one. Our family owned a funeral business for many years back in Minnesota, and I don't think I can remember a time when the hearse wouldn't start," I said, laughing as I turned to enter the reception hall.

Cathy had purchased yellow tablecloths to crisscross over the top of the white linen tablecloths; and she had added yellow flowers to clear glass vases as the centerpiece for each table. She and I organized a tribute table to Mom. We had a picture of mom from when she was fifty years old. We placed our three miniature urns around her picture. At the other end of the table we place a picture of Mom as Mrs. Minnesota and her special memory book. Guests enjoyed looking at her book. Gail and the ladies from the church served cake and refreshments. The large, stark white room seemed cheery as the family greeted old and new friends.

As hard as it was to have Mom pass away, I accepted the fact that it was her time to go. She was ready. In fact, Mom was ready to leave this earth the moment she heard the doctor say, "It's Parkinson's." Her journey had its ups and downs, but we all gained an education along the way. She lived an amazing life, and I feel privileged to have been a part of it.

www.ingramcontent.com/pod-product-compliance
Lightning Source LLC
Chambersburg PA
CBHW051258250726
48656CB00004B/1358